KINESIOLOGY

AN INTRODUCTION TO EXERCISE SCIENCE

Lab Manual & Study Guide

Information on how to obtain copies of this book may be obtained from:

Website: www.thompsonbooks.com
E-mail: publisher@thompsonbooks.com
Telephone: (416) 766-2763
Fax: (416) 766-0398

Library and Archives Canada Cataloguing in Publication

Temertzoglou, Ted, 1964-, author
     Kinesiology : an introduction to exercise science : lab manual
& study guide / Ted Temertozoglou.

ISBN 978-1-55077-234-0 (pbk.)
     1. Kinesiology--Problems, exercises, etc. I. Title.

QP303.T44 2014 Suppl. 1   612.7'6   C2014-906140-4

Publisher: Keith Thompson
Managing Editor: Jane McNulty
Special acknowledgements for their contributions to this edition: Linda Whitmarsh, Durham District School Board, Dave Inglis, Thames Valley District School Board, and Linda Preston, Toronto Catholic District School Board
Editorial Support: Megan Watcher
Cover Design: Gary Blakeley, Blakeley Words+Pictures
Anatomical Illustration: Bart Vallecoccia, B.Sc. AAM (unless otherwise indicated)
Technical Art and Special Effects: Vince Satira

Cover Photos and Credits

Clara Hughes, from Winnipeg, during the women's 3000-metre competition at the World Speedskating Championships in Moscow, Russia, in 2005 (CP Photo/Sergey Ponomarev). Hughes is one of only five people to have podium finishes in the Winter and Summer Olympics, and is the only person ever to have won multiple medals in both.

Justyn Warner competes in the men's 100-metre event at the Canadian Track and Field Championships in Calgary in 2012 (CP Photo/Jeff McIntosh). Justyn attended Middlefield Collegiate Institute and Birchmount Park Collegiate Institute and recently graduated with a B.A. in Kinesiology from Texas Christian University. He was the 2012 Canadian champion in the 100 m and competed in his first Olympic Games in London in 2012. His brother, Ian, was the alternate on the 4x100 m relay team in London.

Vignettes on front cover: Top photo: Canada's Justine Colley, left, drives to the basket during a women's basketball match against Jamaica at the Pan American Games in Guadalajara, Mexico, in 2011 (Ap Photo/Daniel Ochoa de Olza). Middle photo: Canadian snowboarder Michael Lambert makes his way down the men's parallel slalom during qualification runs for the 2014 Winter Olympics in Sochi, Russia (John Lehmann/The Globe and Mail). Bottom photo: Josh Cassidy, from Ottawa, on his way to winning the T53/54 Men's 800-metre wheelchair race during the Paralympic World Cup at the Manchester Regional Arena, Manchester, England, in 2012 (AP Photo/Jon Super).

Vignettes on back cover: Top photo: Canada's Carol Huynh defeats Isabelle Sambou of Senegal to win the bronze medal at the Olympic Games in London, 2012 (CP Photo/Frank Gunn). Bottom photo: A demonstration of Dene games and Arctic sports in Yellowknife, Northwest Territories (PA Photos, 2001).

The publisher and authors wish to thank David J. Sanderson Ph.D. of the UBC Biomechanics Laboratory in the School of Human Kinetics at the University of British Columbia for developing an earlier version of Exercises 13.2 and 13.3, as well as Rowan Thompson, Jeff Claydon, and Kimberlee French, whose photos and video stills appear in Chapters 10 and 13.

Every effort has been made to acquire permission for copyrighted materials used in this book and to acknowledge such permissions accurately. Any errors or omissions called to the publisher's attention will be corrected in future printings.

We acknowledge the support of the Government of Canada through the Canada Book Fund for our publishing activities. We also acknowledge the support of the Government of Ontario through the Ontario Media Development Corporation.

Printed in Canada.
3 4 5 6 7   25 24 23 22 21 20

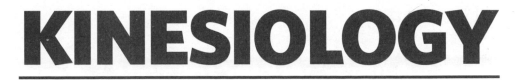

KINESIOLOGY

AN INTRODUCTION TO EXERCISE SCIENCE

LAB MANUAL & STUDY GUIDE

Ted Temertzoglou

THOMPSON EDUCATIONAL PUBLISHING, INC.

Toronto, Ontario

Table of Contents

Introduction

This *Lab Manual & Study Guide* is a "hands-on, minds-on" supplement that supports and, in many cases, expands on the material presented in the student textbook, *Kinesiology: An Introduction to Exercise Science.*

You can think of the exercises in this workbook as "practice sessions" leading up to "game day"—the essays, projects, portfolio work, and examinations that will all contribute to your final mark. The "practice workouts" in this *Lab Manual & Study Guide* will test your knowledge of kinesiology and, it is hoped, encourage you to pursue further studies in the field.

Support for Learning and Assessment

The chapters in the *Lab Manual & Study Guide* align exactly with those in the student textbook. Each activity is designed to enrich your understanding of the chapter and provide opportunities for self-assessment as well as feedback from your teacher and your peers.

- **Learning Goals and Key Terms.** The Learning Goals and Key Terms are reproduced at the beginning of each chapter. Read through them first to refresh your understanding of the content covered in the chapter.

- **Exercises and Lab Activities.** Each chapter contains activities that will enrich your learning through minds-on or hands-on activities, groupwork, observation sessions, and research assignments. They can also be used as a way to assess your understanding of the core content in the textbook.

- **End-of-Chapter Quizzes.** Multiple-choice, short-answer, and brief essay questions are included at the end of each chapter. These provide a quick way to test your understanding of the main ideas in the chapter. Each chapter quiz is divided into two sets, each reviewing the content in roughly half of the chapter.

- **Chapter Review Questions.** The Review Questions at the end of each chapter in the student textbook are reproduced at the end of each chapter in this *Lab Manual & Study Guide*. These questions are subdivided into Achievement Chart assessment categories for easier use by you and your teacher.

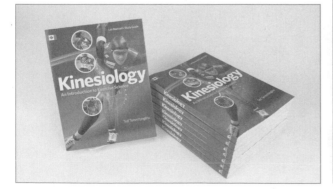

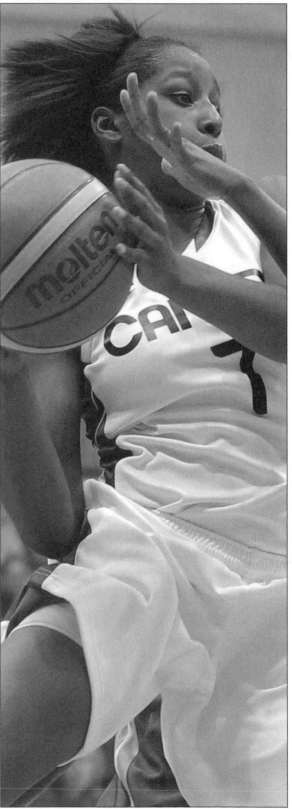

Canada's Justine Colley, left, drives to the basket during a women's basketball match against Jamaica at the Pan American Games in Guadalajara, Mexico, in 2011. (AP Photo/Daniel Ochoa de Olza)

Key Features of this Lab Manual & Study Guide

This *Lab Manual & Study Guide* includes important features that will support you as you encounter the exciting field of kinesiology for the first time:

- **Textbook Preview:** Exercise 1.1 is an overall orientation worksheet that guides you through the structure, organization, text elements, and main features of your kinesiology textbook, while at the same time helping you to clarify your goals in taking this course.

- **Anatomical Drawings for Labelling:** These exercises will provide invaluable support in helping you review and retain terminology related to bones, joints, muscles, energy systems, the heart and blood vessels, and the cardiorespiratory system. The anatomical illustrations in the *Lab Manual & Study Guide* are black-and-white reproductions of the illustrations that appear in the student text but without the labels.

- **CSEP Physical Activity Training for Health (CSEP-PATH) assessment:** The exercises in Chapter 15 replicate some of the assessment tools and fitness tests (updated by the Canadian Society for Exercise Physiology in 2013) that allow qualified exercise professionals to gather information about each client's physical activity, fitness, and lifestyle practices, interpret the findings, and then devise action plans for achieving realistic fitness and wellness goals.

- **Full-Colour Illustrations** are included at the back of this *Lab Manual & Study Guide* for your convenience. Keep these illustrations for future reference, especially if you are thinking of enrolling in a health sciences-related field at college or university.

- **Looking for a Great Career?** Also at the back of this *Lab Manual & Study Guide* are charts that summarize the range of exciting careers available to you in Kinesiology, Physical Education, Recreation and Leisure, and Health Education.

- **Sample Final Exam.** As an added bonus, a Sample Final Exam is provided at the end of this *Lab Manual & Study Guide*. The exam approximates the type of exam your teacher may ask you to take at the end of the course. It is no substitute for studying the material in your student textbook and completing your projects and assignments on time. But it will familiarize you with "game conditions" and help to set you up for success.

Have fun with your kinesiology course. There is no course quite like it, anywhere.

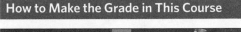

How to Make the Grade in This Course

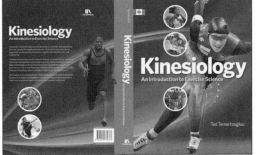

Perhaps it goes without saying: "You will get out of this course exactly what you put into it."

Here are some tips that can help you "make the grade" and have fun at the same time. As you read through the chapters in your textbook, check off the items once you have completed them to your satisfaction.

- ❒ Read through the list of Key Terms and the Learning Goals at the beginning of each chapter in your textbook (they are reproduced in this *Lab Manual & Study Guide* as well). Flag any unfamiliar terminology and be on the lookout for these terms as you progress through the chapter.

- ❒ The Key Terms highlighted throughout the student textbook are defined in the margin and in the Index as well. You may wish to create your own Personal Glossary of Key Terms, enhanced with sketches and mnemonics, to aid comprehension.

- ❒ Re-reading is an effective strategy to strengthen your understanding of material in the student textbook. Re-read material that you found to be complex or unclear on a first read, and flag any sections that might require additional explanation by your teacher.

- ❒ Work on your own, with a "buddy," or in a study group as you record answers to the Chapter Review questions in the textbook and the Chapter Quizzes in this *Lab Manual & Study Guide*.

- ❒ Complete the exercises in this *Lab Manual & Study Guide* with a partner or in a small group. This way you can share ideas and divide up research tasks and note-taking to make them more manageable.

Introducing Kinesiology:
Physical Activity and Sport Today

KEY TERMS

- Mens sana in corpore sano
- Physical inactivity crisis
- Built environment
- Socioeconomic barriers
- Multiculturalism
- Personal and psychological barriers
- Physical literacy
- Long-Term Athlete Development (LTAD)
- Ontario Physical and Health Education Association (Ophea)
- Physical and Health Education Canada (PHE Canada)
- Inclusiveness and accessibility
- Social capital
- Kinesiology
- Lifestyle diseases

A statue of runner Terry Fox in Victoria, B.C. Terry won the 1980 Lou Marsh Award as the nation's top athlete and was named Canada's Newsmaker of the Year. A national hero, he has many buildings, roads, and parks named in his honour.

CP Photo/Don Denton

"Health is a state of complete physical, mental and social well-being and not merely the absence of disease or infirmity."

—The World Health Organization (WHO), Preamble to the Constitution.

The exercises in this chapter of the *Lab Manual & Study Guide* will help to reinforce your understanding of some key concepts and main topics covered in Chapter 1 of your textbook *Kinesiology: An Introduction to Exercise Science.* Along with the Chapter 1 Quiz, these exercises will give you feedback related to the achievement of selected Learning Goals for Chapter 1. For ease of reference, the Chapter 1 Learning Goals from your student textbook are reproduced here:

- describe the correlation between exercise and improved physical and mental well-being
- identify the major contributing factors to global risks to human health and propose possible interventions
- analyze the soaring economic and social costs of inactivity, obesity, and related lifestyle diseases
- describe societal and cultural factors that influence the availability and accessibility of sports and physical activity programs, including the physical literacy movement, the role of educators and role models, and government support
- analyze the individual and social benefits of school and community physical activity and sport programs
- identify ways to overcome barriers to physical activity
- define the discipline of kinesiology and differentiate between academic programs in kinesiology
- identify pathways and opportunities in careers related to kinesiology, physical activity, and sport
- identify prominent Canadians involved in physical activity and sport and describe their contributions

1.1 Preview the Textbook and Clarify Your Learning Goals

Your textbook has been developed to support the curriculum and it will guide your learning in this course. It is worthwhile to take some time to preview its organization, text elements, and main features.

Name: _____

Date: _____

MISSION: Answer the questions below to help you (a) become familiar with the structure of your textbook and (b) clarify your personal learning goals. Once you complete this worksheet, find a partner or a small group with whom to share your answers. Discover whether there are others in your class who share your interests.

1. The organization of your textbook is similar to that of other high school textbooks. Chapter 1, an overview focussing on various "big issues," is followed by four units divided into separate chapters (as shown on the following page). The 16 chapters are followed by a Glossary and an Index at the back of the book. Browse through your textbook's Table of Contents, and then write the titles of Chapters 2 to 16 in the table below. You can abbreviate each title (using one or two words) to fit the spaces provided.

Unit 1: Society, Physical Activity, and Sport	Unit 2: Anatomy and Physiology	Unit 3: Human Performance and Biomechanics	Unit 4: Nutrition, Training, and Ergogenic Aids
2.	5.	9.	14.
3.	6.	10.	15.
4.	7.	11.	16.
	8.	12.	
		13.	

2. Choose a chapter that is of particular interest to you. Find examples of each of the chapter elements listed below. Check each box once you have found that chapter element.
   - ❏ The bulleted lists of Key Terms and Learning Goals at the beginning of the chapter.
   - ❏ The Key Terms highlighted in the text and defined in the margins.
   - ❏ Special two-page "In Focus" features throughout each chapter.
   - ❏ End-of-chapter features (a brief biography of a "Prominent Canadian" or a career profile).
   - ❏ A "Bust a Myth" marginal feature debunking a popular misconception in kinesiology.
   - ❏ The Chapter Review questions at the end of each chapter.

3. Each chapter contains several "In Focus" features. Browse through your textbook's Table of Contents. Select one or two of these "In Focus" features that you find intriguing. Skim the content of these features. Briefly explain why this feature or features caught your attention.

   _____

   _____

   _____

4. Having previewed your textbook's content and organization, answer the following questions: Why did you decide to take this course? Does the course relate to your future goals with respect to education, employment, or enjoyment? (You can refer to the Career Charts on pages 28-29 of the textbook.)

   _____

   _____

   _____

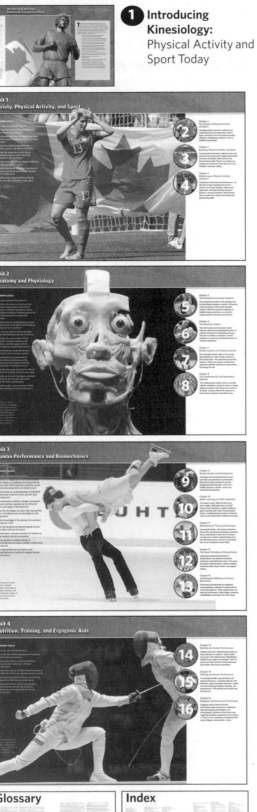

What's Inside Your Textbook?

✔ **Chapter 1—Introduction and Overview**
Chapter 1 introduces several key themes underlying the study of kinesiology today, e.g., the removal of barriers to physical inactivity; the role of schools and communities in promoting healthy, active living; and the scope and benefit of Sport Canada's Long-Term Athlete Development (LTAD) program.

✔ **Four Units (16 Chapters in Total)**
The remaining 15 chapters are grouped into 4 units:
1. Society, Physical Activity, and Sport
2. Anatomy and Physiology
3. Human Performance and Biomechanics
4. Nutrition, Training, and Ergogenic Aids

✔ **Learning Goals**
Curriculum-related Learning Goals are listed at the beginning of each Unit, and more detailed Learning Goals are listed in each chapter opener.

✔ **Anatomical Art, Graphs, Charts, and Photographs**
The text is supported by clearly labelled anatomical illustrations, graphs, charts, and photographs.

✔ **Key Terms Highlighted Throughout the Text**
For easy reference, the Key Terms used in the chapter are listed at the beginning of the chapter. They are also highlighted in the text and defined in the margin.

✔ **Special "In Focus" Features Throughout the Text**
Examples include "Terry Fox: A Canadian Hero"; "Overcoming Racial Barriers in Sport"; "Spinal Cord Injuries and Concussions"; and "What Makes Usain Bolt Run So Fast?"

✔ **"Prominent Canadians" Features**
At the end of selected chapters, there are profiles of Canadians who have made a significant contribution to the world of physical activity and sport.

✔ **Bust A Myth**
These marginal features aim to debunk popular myths related to exercise, nutrition, training, and other relevant topics.

✔ **End-of-Chapter Review**
Each chapter ends with questions categorized according to the provincial Achievement Chart.

✔ **Careers in Kinesiology and Related Fields**
Career Charts in Chapter 1 list the main careers in kinesiology, physical education, recreation and leisure, and health education. "Careers in Focus" features profile Canadians in kinesiology-related fields.

✔ **Glossary of Key Terms**
An alphabetical listing of the key terms along with their definitions can be found at the end of the book.

✔ **Index**
A comprehensive index of key ideas, words, and concepts is also provided at the end of the book.

WORKSHEET

1.2 Physical Inactivity—Removing the Barriers

Many factors contribute to a sedentary lifestyle. This worksheet will help you identify and overcome the barriers that may be undermining your ability to make regular physical activity a part of your daily life.

Name: _____

Date: _____

MISSION: In our hurried and technology-enabled world, sitting rather than moving around is all too common. Barriers to physical activity can be environmental, social, economic, and psychological. Complete the "Barriers to Being Active" Quiz on the following page. Then, use the table below to calculate your score. Finally, refer to the chart on page 14 for help in identifying appropriate strategies to help you overcome the barrier(s) to physical activity that you identified as being especially relevant for you. Grab a pair of comfortable sport shoes, find a workout buddy if you don't like to exercise alone, and put these strategies into action!

Score Yourself on the "Barriers to Being Active" Quiz

Follow these instructions to score yourself:

- In the spaces provided below, enter the number you circled for the applicable question (in the quiz), recording the circled number for Question 1 on row 1, Question 2 on row 2, and so on.
- Add up the three scores in each row. Your barriers to physical activity might fall into one of these categories: lack of time, social influences, lack of energy, lack of motivation, fear of injury, lack of skill, and lack of resources. A score of 5 or above in any category shows that this is an important barrier for you to overcome.

Calculate your score from the quiz on the following page.

_____ + _____ + _____ = _____
(Q1)   (Q8)   (Q15)   **Lack of time**

_____ + _____ + _____ = _____
(Q2)   (Q9)   (Q16)   **Social influences**

_____ + _____ + _____ = _____
(Q3)   (Q10)   (Q17)   **Lack of energy**

_____ + _____ + _____ = _____
(Q4)   (Q11)   (Q18)   **Lack of motivation**

_____ + _____ + _____ = _____
(Q5)   (Q12)   (Q19)   **Fear of injury**

_____ + _____ + _____ = _____
(Q6)   (Q13)   (Q20)   **Lack of skill**

_____ + _____ + _____ = _____
(Q7)   (Q14)   (Q21)   **Lack of resources**

TOTAL SCORE [_____]

Source: Adapted from "Barriers to Physical Activity Quiz." In *Physical Activity for Everyone: Overcoming Barriers to Physical Activity* (Centers for Disease Control and Prevention).

"Barriers to Being Active" Quiz

Listed below are reasons that people commonly give to describe why they do not get as much physical activity as they think they should. Read each statement and then indicate how likely you are to say each one. Circle the applicable number for each statement—"3" means "very likely" and "0" means "not likely at all."

How likely are you to say...?				
1. My day is so busy now, I just don't think I can make the time to include physical activity in my regular schedule.	3	2	1	0
2. None of my family members or friends likes to do anything active, so I don't have a chance to exercise.	3	2	1	0
3. I'm just too tired after school or work to get any exercise.	3	2	1	0
4. I've been thinking about getting more exercise, but I just can't seem to get started.	3	2	1	0
5. Exercise can be risky.	3	2	1	0
6. I don't get enough exercise because I have never learned the skills for any sport.	3	2	1	0
7. I don't have access to jogging trails, swimming pools, bike paths, etc.	3	2	1	0
8. Physical activity takes too much time away from other commitments—school, work, family, etc.	3	2	1	0
9. I'm embarrassed about how I will look when I exercise with others.	3	2	1	0
10. I don't get enough sleep as it is. I just couldn't get up early or stay up late to get some exercise.	3	2	1	0
11. It's easier for me to find excuses not to exercise than to go out to do something.	3	2	1	0
12. I know of too many people who have hurt themselves by overdoing it with exercise.	3	2	1	0
13. I really can't see learning a new sport.	3	2	1	0
14. It's just too expensive. You have to take a class or join a club or buy the right equipment.	3	2	1	0
15. My free times during the day are too short to include exercise.	3	2	1	0
16. My usual social activities with family or friends do not include physical activity.	3	2	1	0
17. I'm too tired during the week and I need the weekend to catch up on my rest.	3	2	1	0
18. I want to get more exercise, but I just can't seem to make myself stick to anything.	3	2	1	0
19. I'm afraid I might injure myself.	3	2	1	0
20. I'm not good enough at any physical activity to make it fun.	3	2	1	0
21. If we had exercise facilities and showers at school or at work, then I would be more likely to exercise.	3	2	1	0

Overcoming Barriers to Physical Activity

Barriers	Suggested Strategies for Overcoming Barriers
Lack of time	• Identify the available time slots or create time slots during which you are willing to give up a sedentary activity (e.g., watching television). Monitor your daily activities for one week. Identify at least three 30-minute time slots you could use for physical activity. • Add physical activity to your daily routine (e.g., walk or ride your bike to school, work, or shopping malls, organize school activities around physical activity, walk the dog, exercise while you watch TV, park farther away from your destination). • Make time for physical activity (e.g., walk, jog, or swim during your lunch hour, take fitness breaks while you study, walk up and down stairs between classes). • Select activities requiring minimal time, such as walking, jogging, or stair climbing.
Social influences	• Explain your interest in physical activity to friends and family. Ask them to support your efforts. • Invite friends and family members to exercise with you. Plan social activities involving exercise. • Develop new friendships with physically active people. Join a group (e.g., a hiking or cycling club).
Lack of energy	• Schedule physical activity for times in the day or week when you feel energetic. • Convince yourself that if you give it a chance, physical activity will increase your energy level; then, try it.
Lack of motivation	• Plan ahead and make the commitment. Make physical activity a regular part of your daily or weekly schedule and write it on your calendar. • Invite a friend to exercise with you on a regular basis and write it on both your calendars. • Join an exercise group or class.
Fear of injury	• Learn how to warm up and cool down to prevent injury. • Learn how to exercise appropriately, considering your age, fitness level, skill level, and health status. • Choose activities involving minimal risk.
Lack of skill	• Select activities requiring no new skills, such as walking, climbing stairs, or jogging. • Exercise with friends who are at the same skill level as you are. • Find a friend who is willing to teach you some new skills. • Take a class to develop new skills.
Lack of resources	• Select activities that require minimal facilities or equipment, such as walking, jogging, jumping rope, calisthenics, yoga, or Pilates. • Identify inexpensive, convenient resources available in your community (e.g., community education programs, park and recreation programs, worksite programs).
Weather conditions	• Develop a set of regular activities that are always available regardless of weather (e.g., indoor cycling, aerobic dance, indoor swimming, calisthenics, stair climbing, jumping rope, mall walking, dancing, gymnasium games). • Look on outdoor activities that depend on weather conditions (e.g., cross-country skiing, snowshoeing, skating, outdoor swimming, outdoor tennis) as "bonuses"—extra activities possible when weather and circumstances permit.
Travel	• Put a jumping rope in your suitcase and use it whenever you can. • Walk the halls and climb the stairs in hotels. • Stay in places with swimming pools or exercise facilities. • Join the YMCA or YWCA (ask about a reciprocal membership agreement). • During gas station stops, take exercise breaks. • Bring your favourite music that motivates you.
Family involvement	• Exercise with your brother or sister when babysitting (e.g., go for a walk together, play tag or other running games, get an aerobic dance DVD for kids and exercise together). You can spend time together and still get your exercise. • Find ways to be active around your home with others (e.g., shoot hoops, play tennis at a nearby tennis court, go for a bicycle ride with a friend, play with siblings, do household chores such as sweeping floors or mowing the lawn).

Source: Centers for Disease Control and Prevention. 2007. "Overcoming Barriers to Physical Activity."
Physical Activity for Everyone.

WORKSHEET

1.3 Physical Literacy: What's It All About?

Just as we need to learn reading, writing, and math, we need to learn to move confidently and to understand the social contexts of physical activity, sport, and healthy living. Everyone needs to become "physically literate."

Name: _____

Date: _____

Concept maps allow you to organize a set of related ideas in a visual way. You can use words, diagrams, and pictures to represent your ideas and how they are related to each other. This worksheet asks you to create a concept map on the following page that represents the various components and benefits of physical literacy.

You can then consolidate your ideas and compose your own personal definition of "physical literacy."

(A) Thinking about Physical Literacy

MISSION: Represent the basic meaning as well as the personal and social implications of physical literacy by creating a Physical Literacy Concept Map on the following page.

Once you have itemized the key components and benefits of physical literacy, compose your own personal definition that you can refer to during this course. Write your definition in the space provided on the following page.

Use the following questions to prompt your thinking:

1. How does your textbook define "physical literacy"?

2. How can individuals of varying ages and abilities gain and maintain competence in movement?

3. Why is confidence in movement an important component of physical literacy? Why might someone lack the confidence to move? What are the implications for individuals who do not have confidence in their ability to move?

4. Why is it important to be able to move in a wide variety of environments in Canada?

5. How does being physically literate benefit the whole person? Think of all the possible benefits of being physically literate.

6. Of what importance is physical literacy to Canada's Long-Term Athlete Development (LTAD) model?

7. What impact does physical literacy have upon you? Your school? Your community? Your nation?

(B) Follow-up Activities

MISSION: Once you have completed your concept map, choose one, some, or all of these follow-up activities to complete, either on your own or in a group, according to your teacher's instructions.

1. As a class, brainstorm a list of people who could be described as "physically literate." Be sure that they represent all or most aspects of the definition of physical literacy. These individuals may be from your school, community, or country. In what ways do they personify physical literacy?

2. Create a small poster or a one-page newsletter article about someone that you consider to be a "Physical Literacy Champion." Include a photograph of the individual and descriptions or visuals of the activities that your champion likes to pursue. Summarize why this person is an excellent role model.

3. Create a collage showing in what ways you are a physically literate individual. Along with your collage, write a short paragraph that describes you and why you consider yourself to be physically literate. Refer to the visuals in your collage as examples to support your writing. What more could you do to keep improving your physical literacy?

4. With your classmates, brainstorm how your class and/or school could support the improvement of physical literacy in your school, feeder schools, and community in general. What practical steps could you take to implement one or more of the ideas proposed?

PHYSICAL LITERACY CONCEPT MAP

_____

Physical literacy is related to...

_____

_____

_____

_____

_____

_____

My Personal Definition of "Physical Literacy"

_____

_____

_____

_____

_____

_____

_____

WORKSHEET

1.4 What Is Kinesiology?

Over the past 50 years or so, kinesiology has been the fastest growing discipline at colleges and universities. The study of kinesiology can provide a strong entry point to a lifelong career in many fascinating fields.

Name: _____

Date: _____

MISSION: In this exercise, you are encouraged to expand the concept map below that represents the components of kinesiology as a field of study. (The graphic is the same as the one on page 25 in your textbook.) On the lines provided, jot down topics related to each component of the field of kinesiology. Feel free to refer to your textbook to check to see whether your suggested topics are directly related to the discipline of kinesiology.

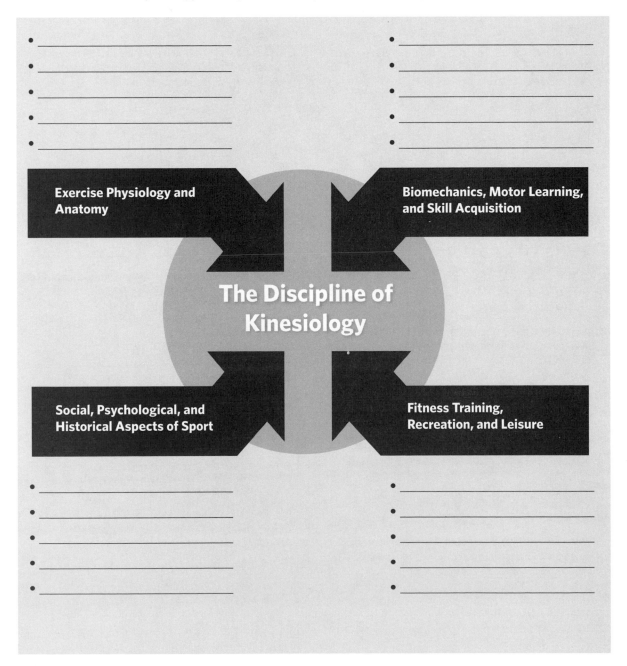

- _____
- _____
- _____
- _____
- _____

- _____
- _____
- _____
- _____
- _____

Exercise Physiology and Anatomy

Biomechanics, Motor Learning, and Skill Acquisition

The Discipline of Kinesiology

Social, Psychological, and Historical Aspects of Sport

Fitness Training, Recreation, and Leisure

- _____
- _____
- _____
- _____
- _____

- _____
- _____
- _____
- _____
- _____

WORKSHEET

Chapter 1 Quiz

The two sets of questions below will test your knowledge and broaden your understanding of the material covered in Chapter 1. Complete each set of questions according to your teacher's instructions.

Name: _____

Date: _____

Question Set 1: Inactivity and Obesity—Overcoming the Barriers

Multiple-Choice Questions

MISSION: Circle the letter beside the answer that you believe to be correct.

1. The Latin expression *Mens sana in corpore sano* means
   (a) an agile mind in an athletic body
   (b) a clear mind in a muscular body
   (c) a wise mind in an aging body
   (d) a sound mind in a healthy body

2. Dr. John Ratey and other brain researchers have demonstrated that physical activity
   (a) increases energy levels
   (b) enhances mood
   (c) improves memory
   (d) all of the above

3. Insufficient physical activity around the world is associated with
   (a) increased morbidity and mortality worldwide
   (b) decreased industrial safety worldwide
   (c) a declining birth rate worldwide
   (d) lower income levels worldwide

4. What is the basic physical activity target for adults in Canada in terms of moderate to vigorous exercise per week?
   (a) 75 minutes
   (b) 150 minutes
   (c) 250 minutes
   (d) 100 minutes

5. The ratio of a person's weight in kilograms to the square of his or her height in metres is known as
   (a) DALYs
   (b) CAD
   (c) BMI
   (d) MRI

6. One of the main culprits contributing to lifestyle diseases in industrialized countries, as identified by the World Health Organization, is
   (a) sedentarism
   (b) air pollution
   (c) autoimmune deficiency
   (d) overreliance on prescription drugs

Short-Answer Questions

MISSION: Briefly answer the following questions in the space provided:

1. List some ways in which daily life in developed nations has reduced people's opportunities to expend physical energy.

2. What is meant by the "built environment"?

3. What three recommended behavioural changes can prevent most lifestyle diseases?

Essay Questions

MISSION: On a separate piece of paper, develop a 100-word response to the following questions.

1. Discuss the effects of physical activity on mental performance.

2. Explain why health experts believe that the physical inactivity crisis is threatening the health of multiple generations of Canadians.

3. Describe and evaluate the most effective ways to overcome barriers to physical activity.

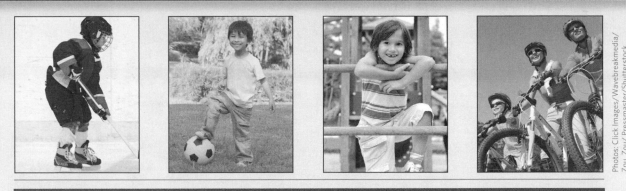

Photos: Click Images/Wavebreakmedia/ Zou Zou/ Pressmaster/Shutterstock

Question Set 2: Physical Literacy and the Study of Kinesiology

Multiple-Choice Questions

MISSION: Circle the letter beside the answer that you believe to be correct.

1. The key to physical literacy lies in
   (a) more funding for Canadian Sport Centres
   (b) publicity campaigns to promote healthy living
   (c) tax breaks for parents or guardians who enrol their children in recreational programs
   (d) strong physical education programs at the school level

2. The main focus of amateur hockey leagues is
   (a) learning team skills
   (b) teaching athletes to have fun
   (c) improving the competitive level of the sport
   (d) supporting amateur hockey in Canada

3. The benefits of community sport and physical activity programs include
   (a) reduced smoking, drug use, and alcohol consumption
   (b) support services for at-risk youth and newcomers to Canada
   (c) decreased incidence of illness and injury
   (d) all of the above

4. Sport and recreation create what sociologists refer to as
   (a) human capital
   (b) physical capital
   (c) social capital
   (d) monetary benefits

5. According to the Long-Term Athlete Development (LTAD) model, children do best when they engage in activities that suit their
   (a) developmental level
   (b) grade level
   (c) chronological age
   (d) height and weight

6. The LTAD model focusses on
   (a) Canadian national sport policy
   (b) a training, competition, and recovery pathway
   (c) intramural sports
   (d) amateur athletics

Short-Answer Questions

MISSION: Briefly answer the following questions in the space provided:

1. Name at least three national and provincial organizations that are spearheading the physical literacy campaign in schools.

2. Name the apparently harmless act that has been described as a "deadly killer in our midst."

3. List four different occupational areas associated with a degree or diploma in kinesiology.

Essay Questions

MISSION: On a separate piece of paper, develop a 100-word response to the following questions.

1. Discuss ways to reduce concerns about children's safety in order to boost participation in informal games and unstructured activities in playgrounds, fields, and parks.

2. Explain how Canadian Sport for Life's Long-Term Athlete Development (LTAD) model is one of its most important cornerstones.

3. What are some ways to enter the field of kinesiology?

WORKSHEET

My Notes on Chapter 1

Use the space below to make notes on the questions on the facing page, to record any thoughts and ideas you have on this chapter, and to store study tips to help you prepare for tests and exams.

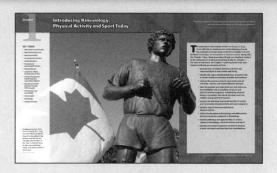

Chapter 1 Review (Student Textbook page 31)

Knowledge

1. Describe at least four ways in which physical activity can enhance mental performance, as shown by medical researchers such as Dr. John Ratey.

2. List as many benefits as you can that are associated with regular participation in physical exercise or sport. Compare your list with one generated by another student and note similarities and differences.

3. How many minutes per week do you spend in moderate to vigorous exercise, and do you meet the basic target recommended by Canadian health experts? If you have younger siblings, do they meet the recommended target for children between the ages of five and 17? Elaborate on your answer.

4. Distinguish between direct and indirect health-care costs resulting from insufficient levels of physical activity in Canada.

5. What is physical literacy, why is it important, and how is physical literacy promoted in schools and communities across Canada?

6. Differentiate between "fun leagues" and organized sports leagues for children and youth. Describe some advantages and disadvantages of each type of league.

7. Why would kinesiology be a good program of study for someone who enjoys variety and a multi-disciplinary approach?

Thinking and Inquiry

8. Identify what you perceive as the top three most serious health risks related to physical inactivity in your community. Suggest ways to combat these risks.

9. Technologies such as television, computers, video games, smartphones, tablets, and other digital devices have contributed to the inactivity crisis because they lend themselves to sedentary behaviours. Suggest ways to encourage children and teenagers to balance or replace their sedentary pastimes with regular physical recreation.

10. Do you think the provincial and federal governments should provide tax breaks (incentives) to companies that offer health and wellness programs or gym memberships to their employees as part of their benefits package? Why or why not?

11. Suggest strategies by which obese or overweight individuals and families can be encouraged to achieve a healthier body weight in ways that do not cause them shame, fear, or embarrassment.

12. Draw a Venn diagram to show how the benefits of school health and physical education programs overlap with the benefits of community sport and physical activity programs.

13. Why do you think our educational and health-care systems find it difficult to ensure that students are physically active for at least one hour a day?

14. Kinesiology has become one of the fastest growing fields of research and study at colleges and universities over the past 50 years. What accounts for this?

Communication

15. Browse through recent print and/or online materials that discuss the worldwide physical inactivity crisis. Summarize the authors' findings in a table under the following three headings: (1) Country, Region, or City; (2) Causes of Insufficient Physical Activity; and (3) Possible Interventions. After completing the table, briefly present your findings orally in class.

16. Devise a slogan and a four-point plan for a community public awareness campaign to encourage people to eat a healthier diet and to get more exercise.

17. Draw a simple diagram to show possible academic and career pathways followed by someone who wishes to become (a) a ski instructor; (b) a play therapist; and (c) a personal trainer.

Application

18. Would you recommend that the Canadian Medical Association change its thinking and declare obesity to be a disease rather than a lifestyle issue? State reasons why or why not.

19. Review the seven stages of Canadian Sport for Life's Long-Term Athlete Development Model. Match each member of your family, including yourself, to one of the seven stages, and explain your reasoning.

20. Describe the attributes of a mentor or role model who has helped you become more physically literate.

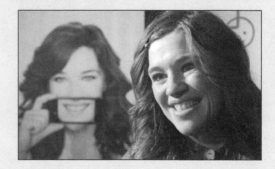

Canadian Olympic athlete Clara Hughes speaks during an announcement in Ottawa, September 21, 2010. Bell Canada announced it would invest $64 million in mental health initiatives. (CP Photo/Adrian Wyld)

The History of Physical Activity and Sport

KEY TERMS

- Olympic Games
- Athleticism
- Renaissance man
- Industrial Revolution
- Amateurism
- Modern Olympic Games
- Nationalism
- Olympic truce
- Professional sports
- Sports franchise
- American Civil War
- Feminine ideal
- Title IX
- Sport Canada
- ParticipACTION
- Canadian Sport Policy 2012
- Canadian Olympic Committee (COC)
- Own the Podium

Canada's Carol Huynh defeats Isabelle Sambou of Senegal to win the bronze medal at the Olympic Games in London, 2012. Dropped as an Olympic sport in February 2013, wrestling was reinstated for the 2020 Olympics following a backlash.

CP Photo/Frank Gunn

The exercises in this chapter of the *Lab Manual & Study Guide* will help to reinforce your understanding of some key concepts and main topics covered in Chapter 2 of your textbook *Kinesiology: An Introduction to Exercise Science.* Along with the Chapter 2 Quiz, these exercises will give you feedback related to the achievement of selected Learning Goals for Chapter 2. For ease of reference, the Chapter 2 Learning Goals from your student textbook are reproduced here:

• describe the historical evolution of physical activity and sport in the context of changing societal and cultural values

• describe factors that influence participation in physical activity and sport, e.g., gender or socioeconomic status

• analyze the role that sport has played in various cultures and societies from early human history to present day

• describe some unique contributions of Aboriginal peoples in the Americas to physical activity and sport

• analyze the changing relationships between Olympic ideals, nationalism, and global politics

• identify the social and historical factors that contributed to the rise of professional sports leagues in North America

• identify historical landmarks and pioneers in the removal of gender and racial barriers in sport and physical activity

• examine historical developments in Canadian government sport policy/organization and support for physical literacy

• describe societal and cultural factors that influence the availability and accessibility of sport and physical activity

• identify prominent Canadians involved in physical activity and sport and describe their contributions

• identify career opportunities in fields related to physical activity and sport

WORKSHEET

2.1 Sporting Values—An Historical Timeline

Physical activity and sport are intricately linked to society as a whole. The predominant societal attitudes and values of a specific time period are often reflected in the sporting values of that period as well.

Name: _____

Date: _____

MISSION: Demonstrate your understanding of the relationship between societal values and sporting values in three different historical time periods.

Fill in the timeline chart on these two pages to the best of your ability, and then answer the discussion questions that appear at the top of the next page.

	1. The Early Period: Ancient Greeks and Romans
1. Describe the social significance of physical activity and sport during this time period. What main purposes or roles did physical activity and sport fulfill for society?	
2. What would you say were the predominant societal values that characterized this time period?	
3. What would you say were the predominant sporting values that characterized this time period?	
4. How equitable was access to physical activity and sport as leisure pursuits during this time period? Explain your answer.	

Discussion Questions

1. There is a clear connection between societal values and sporting values. Do you think that societal values are reflected in sporting values, or vice-versa? Explain using examples.

2. As Western society has evolved, do you perceive an increase or a decrease in access to physical activity and sport? Give examples of social groups that had and did not have access to sport and physical activity in the past.

3. What important societal values do you think can be reinforced through sport today? Where do you see societal values and sporting values shifting in the future?

4. How can international sport competitions, such as the Olympics, help to promote a greater understanding of the cultures and values of other nations? What importance do these events hold for world societies?

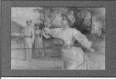 **2. The Industrial Revolution and the Victorian Era**

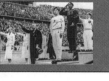 **3. The Modern Period (The 1896 Olympics and Beyond)**

2.2 Canadian Sport Heroes and Their Achievements

Understanding the historical context of physical activity and sport can deepen your insights into current trends and events. This exercise acquaints you with contributions made by Canadians in the history of sport.

Name: _____

Date: _____

MISSION: Research the major achievements of the following Canadian sport figures, and fill in the table below.

Athlete	Major Achievements
James Naismith 1891	
Tom Longboat 1905 –1915	
Barbara Ann Scott 1940s	
Abigail Hoffman 1950s –1970s	
Dick Pound 1960s	
Arnie Boldt 1960s –1970s	

Nancy Greene 1960s – 1970s	
Wayne Gretzky 1980s – 1990s	
Hayley Wickenheiser 1990s – present	
Chantal Petitclerc 1990s – present	
Cindy Klassen 2000 – 2012	
Alexandre Bilodeau 2006 – 2014	
[Your own sport hero]	

WORKSHEET

2.3 The Canadian Sport Community

The sport community in Canada consists of a number of organizations that provide sport programming and activities at the municipal, provincial/territorial, national, and international levels.

Name: _____

Date: _____

(A) The Sport Community in Canada

MISSION: This assignment will familiarize you with the major sport organizations in Canada. These organizations are responsible for providing sport programming at various levels.

Complete the following chart using a minimum of three examples for each level of sport indicated. Where the organization has a website, indicate the URL and other information that the website provides.

Local	Provincial	National	International
Local or community sport clubs	Provincial Games Organizations	National Games Organizations	Major Games Federations
School clubs and teams	Provincial Sport Organizations	National Sport Organizations	International Sport Federations
Post-secondary institutions' clubs/ teams	Provincial Multi-Sport Organizations	National Multi-Sport Organizations	General Assemblies of International Sports

(B) Provincial Sport Organizations (PSOs)

MISSION: Provincial Sport Organizations (PSOs) play an important role in providing opportunities for physical activity and sport for Canadians. To gain an understanding of how Provincial Sport Organizations operate, choose and research a Provincial Sport Organization and then fill in the chart below.

Full name of PSO, location, and website address	
Year in which the PSO was founded	
Number of local clubs represented	
Total current individual members—is the membership growing?	
Number of full-time staff	
Annual total expenditure of the PSO	
Amount of funding received in most recent year	
Current programs offered by the PSO	
Significant past achievements of the PSO	
Future goals of the PSO	

Chapter 2 Quiz

The two sets of questions below will test your knowledge and broaden your understanding of the material covered in Chapter 2. Complete each set of questions according to your teacher's instructions.

Name: _____

Date: _____

Question Set 1: From Ancient Times to the Revival of the Modern Olympics (1896)

Multiple-Choice Questions

MISSION: Circle the letter beside the answer that you believe to be correct.

1. Which civilization first articulated how physical activity can benefit the mind as well as the body?
   (a) the Aztecs
   (b) the ancient Greeks
   (c) the ancient Romans
   (d) the Europeans of the Renaissance

2. Physical education classes for children were instituted in 1420 in Europe by
   (a) Leonardo da Vinci
   (b) Pierre de Coubertin
   (c) Queen Victoria
   (d) Italian physician Vittorino da Feltre

3. The Victorian gentleman athlete embraced the concept of
   (a) fair play
   (b) amateurism
   (c) sport as a reflection of life
   (d) all of the above

4. Which cultural group invented lacrosse?
   (a) Early French settlers in the New World
   (b) the Aztecs
   (c) Ancient Greek warriors
   (d) Aboriginal peoples of North America

5. What does the term "Olympic truce" mean?
   (a) offerings all athletes have to bring in order to be allowed to compete
   (b) ceremonial clothing worn by early Olympians
   (c) a global and symbolic agreement aimed at promoting friendly relations between nations
   (d) the prize offered to victorious athletes in early Olympic competition

6. In 2002, the Paralympic Games achieved a major breakthrough in public awareness
   (a) through the efforts of Dr. Robert F. Jackson
   (b) when Canada ranked amongst the top nations
   (c) when highlights were aired on the A&E cable network in the U.S. and on CBC in Canada
   (d) because the Games were held in Salt Lake City

Short-Answer Questions

MISSION: Briefly answer the following questions in the space provided:

1. Did Greek and Roman concepts of sport have any effect on each other? If so, what was it?

2. Why was the concept of "athleticism" embraced again during the Renaissance?

3. Why did the Victorians believe that participation in sports was harmful to women?

Essay Questions

MISSION: On a separate piece of paper, develop a 100-word response to the following questions.

1. Elaborate on the evolving social significance of sports to Aboriginal peoples in North America.

2. Analyze the relationship between nationalism and sport as demonstrated by the goals of the modern Olympic Games.

3. Explain why the principle of "equal access" to physical activity and sport is an important value in Canadian society.

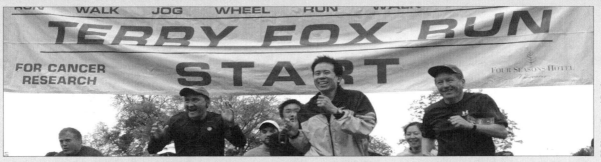

CP Photo/Darryl Dyck

Question Set 2: The Modern History of Physical Activity and Sport (1900-Present)

Multiple-Choice Questions

MISSION: Circle the letter beside the answer that you believe to be correct.

1. Professional sport competition arose when
   (a) amateurism was no longer valued
   (b) teams started paying their best players to retain them full-time and to motivate them
   (c) Olympic sports became less popular
   (d) the Victorian age was at its height

2. The only fully professional major women's sports league in North America is
   (a) the Women's National Hockey Association
   (b) the Women's National Soccer Association
   (c) the Women's National Basketball Association
   (d) the Women's National Curling Association

3. The emergence of the modern sports fan began as a result of
   (a) the rise of the Internet
   (b) industrialization and increased leisure time, including time to read about sports heroes
   (c) the aftermath of the American Civil War
   (d) changing attitudes towards women in sports

4. No women competed in the first modern Olympic Games in 1896 because many people believed that
   (a) women were more athletic than men
   (b) women were too afraid to compete
   (c) a "woman's place" was in the home
   (d) a "woman's place" was in the factory

5. Sport Canada, the major granting agency for sports in Canada, is located within
   (a) the Athlete Assistance Program
   (b) each provincial and territorial government
   (c) the Department of Canadian Heritage
   (d) the community of National Games Organizations

6. A driving force behind Canada's evolution into a world-leading sport organization is
   (a) Athletics Canada
   (b) Own the Podium
   (c) International Amateur Athletics Federation
   (d) Tennis Canada

Short-Answer Questions

MISSION: Briefly answer the following questions in the space provided:

1. Outline the primary goals of Sport Canada and the Canadian Sport Policy 2012.

2. What is the main responsibility of the Canadian Olympic Committee?

3. Who were the Edmonton Grads and what were the keys to their success?

Essay Questions

MISSION: On a separate piece of paper, develop a 100-word response to the following questions.

1. Explain how the history of women's participation in sport has involved changing societal attitudes and the destruction of stereotypes.

2. Describe how the history of international sport reflects a struggle against exclusionary practices towards various ethnic groups.

3. Describe ways in which the Canadian government and the sport community in Canada promote active, healthy living.

My Notes on Chapter 2

Use the space below to make notes on the questions on the facing page, to record any thoughts and ideas you have on this chapter, and to store study tips to help you prepare for tests and exams.

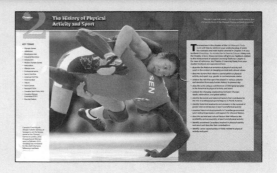

_____

_____

_____

_____

_____

_____

_____

_____

_____

_____

_____

_____

_____

_____

_____

_____

_____

_____

_____

_____

_____

_____

_____

_____

Chapter 2 Review (Student Textbook page 65)

Knowledge

1. Describe how the concept of what it means to be an athlete has changed from the time of the ancient Greeks and Romans to the present.
2. Which social groups did the Victorian ideal of the amateur athlete include and exclude from participating in organized sports and games, and why?
3. What roles have sports played in Aboriginal societies in the Americas? Give two specific examples.
4. What social and historical factors contributed to the rise of professional sports leagues in North America?
5. Identify five Canadian sports pioneers who overcame racial barriers in order to participate in their chosen sport, and state their accomplishments.
6. Describe how societal attitudes towards "women's place" in sport have changed since the Victorian era, drawing parallels to the evolution of women's rights in areas other than sport and physical activity.
7. Identify some goals, policies, and initiatives by means of which our federal government's Department of Canadian Heritage, through Sport Canada, seeks to promote sport and physical activity for all Canadians.

Thinking and Inquiry

8. Choose a sport featured in the Paralympics and research how technology has made an impact on that sport. Summarize your findings in a brief report.
9. Should a country that allegedly violates international treaties such as those designed to protect human rights be allowed to participate in today's Olympic Games? Discuss this issue as a class or in a small group.
10. If you could interview a Canadian sports pioneer who struggled to break either the gender barrier or the colour barrier, what key question or questions would you ask that person? Do some research to try to learn more about that individual.
11. Why are the terms "inclusion" and "equality" important key words when reviewing the history of sport and physical activity in Canadian society?
12. In what ways might the various ministries and organizations responsible for implementing sport policy in Canada measure the effectiveness of the Canadian Sport Policy 2012 in achieving its goals?

Communication

13. In a graphic organizer such as a timeline, a table, or a flow chart, show how the Olympic Games have changed from their revival in 1896 to the present day. Include some changes in countries, sports, participants, and sporting rules.
14. Choose your favourite sports league and show its origins and some selected historical highlights in a timeline. Include illustrations if you wish.
15. Choose a female role model and write a brief profile explaining how that individual changed social perceptions of women's place in sport and physical activity.
16. Write and present a brief analysis of a recent incident of racism related to sport as reported in national or international media. Discuss public response to the incident in class.
17. Create a slideshow or a poster depicting how changes in the concept of "athleticism" have both reflected and influenced Western societal values over time.

Application

18. Do you think that the Roman concept of "a sound mind in a sound body" is as important today as it was in ancient times? Explain your answer.
19. Journalists and media commentators sometimes refer to the social ideal of the "Renaissance man" or "Renaissance woman" to describe a certain type of individual today. Compare and contrast the original concept with today's concept.
20. Suppose that Title IX legislation had not been passed in the United States. How might that have affected girls' and women's participation in sport in Canada?
21. Identify a modern female sports team or delegation, who, like the Edmonton Grads, have served as ambassadors for Canada on the world stage. Briefly describe their accomplishments.
22. In a group, discuss examples of Canadian federal government initiatives to promote active, healthy living that are evident in your school or community. Evaluate the effectiveness of these initiatives in terms of specific criteria that you decide on as a group.

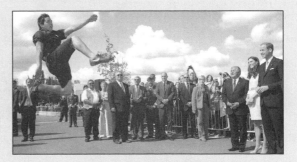

A demonstration of Dene games and Arctic sports in Yellowknife, Northwest Territories. PA Photos, 2001

Business, Physical Activity, and Sport

KEY TERMS

- Professional athlete
- Amateur athlete
- Endorsement
- Athlete Assistance Program
- For-profit sport
- Not-for-profit sport
- Sport franchise
- Sports agent
- Media
- Broadcasting rights
- Social media
- Private fitness industry

Fans wait out a blackout prior to the start of an NHL game between the Edmonton Oilers and Ottawa Senators, at Edmonton's Rexall Place.

Ververidis Vasilis/Shutterstock

The exercises in this chapter of the *Lab Manual & Study Guide* will help to reinforce your understanding of some key concepts and main topics covered in Chapter 3 of your textbook *Kinesiology: An Introduction to Exercise Science.* Along with the Chapter 3 Quiz, these exercises will give you feedback related to the achievement of selected Learning Goals for Chapter 3. For ease of reference, the Chapter 3 Learning Goals from your student textbook are reproduced here:

- analyze the relationships between business, physical activity, and sport

- differentiate between professional and amateur athletes

- analyze sport as a profit-making enterprise that relies on various revenue streams and spin-off ventures

- identify the roles and rewards of key players in sport: owners, agents, players, and fans

- analyze issues related to salaries, endorsements, and funding in both professional and amateur sport

- analyze issues related to sport as entertainment, e.g., broadcasting rights and ownership concentration

- analyze the influence of TV and other media, including social media, on sport and physical activity

- identify some historical and social factors contributing to the emergence of the modern sports fan

- explain the importance of being an informed consumer with regard to physical activity and sport

- describe ways in which consumers of health and fitness products and services can protect themselves

- identify career opportunities in fields related to physical activity and sport

- identify prominent Canadians involved in physical activity and sport and describe their contributions

WORKSHEET

3.1 Contrasting Viewpoints on the Business of Sport

Athletes, agents, team owners, and broadcasters benefit from the large sums of money generated by professional sports events, but certain trends in the "big business" of sport may benefit some more than others.

Name: _____

Date: _____

MISSION: Complete the chart below with one of three responses: "PRO," "CON," or "NR" ("not relevant"). If you respond "PRO" or "CON," provide a rationale to support your opinion.

Your viewpoint will depend on whether you think that athletes/agents, team owners, sports fans, or broadcasters would be in favour of the sport trend indicated. A sample entry is provided below.

	Athletes/Agents	Team Owners	Sports Fans	Broadcasters
"In general, ticket prices for sports events need to be higher."	PRO—expectation that increased revenue will lead to higher player salaries	PRO—expectation of increased revenue	CON—becomes harder for average fan to attend events	NR—Price of live admission is irrelevant to broadcaster
"There needs to be more advertising on televised events."				
"Players' unions need to be strengthened."				
"Top players' salaries are still too low."				
"Spin-off products are overpriced because it is extremely costly to operate a sport franchise."				

☞ Look in the Book, pp. 80-83; p. 88

WORKSHEET

3.2 Changes Inspired in Sport by Television

Of the various forms of media, television has had the most influential impact on the world of sport. Entire games are now "timed" to align with potential television advertising revenues based on ratings and numbers of viewers.

Name: ______________________________

Date: ______________________________

MISSION: For each sport indicated in the chart below, list a fundamental change that occurred due to the influences of television coverage and/or the advertising that accompanies it. Changes can include: rules of the sport, the redesign of uniforms and/or equipment worn/used by the athletes, or even the duration and tempo of the sporting event. A sample entry is provided below.

Sport	Impact/Change Factor	When
NBA (Basketball)	"TV Time-outs" held approximately every 4 minutes to allow for more commercials during telecasts	1990s
NFL/CFL Football		
NHL Hockey		
Soccer		
Boxing (Pro or Amateur)		
Pro Golf		
Auto Racing		
Pro Baseball		
Pro Tennis		
Track and Field		

WORKSHEET

3.3 The "Lions' Den" and the Sport Consumer

The marketing of goods and services related to sports and physical activity is a booming business. Consumers want value for their money, and they expect (or hope) that their purchase will deliver positive results.

Name: _____

Date: _____

MISSION: With a partner or in a small group, use the template on the facing page to draw up a business proposal for a product or service that would offer value for someone involved in physical activity or sport.

When you have completed your proposal, you will present it in a simulated "Lions' Den" for feedback. (The "Lions" can be either a panel of students selected from the class or the class as a whole.)

The "Lions" will judge the feasibility of your proposed product or service objectively against the 10-point feasibility criteria outlined in the chart below. In their role as judges, they will show no favouritism.

The "Lions' Den" panel will decide which proposal will receive their financial backing. If you are on the Lions' Den panel, be prepared to defend your decisions. Good luck!

Making an Investment Decision — Lions' Score Card (Criteria)	Out of 10 points
1. Has the proposal described the features of the product or service in adequate detail for an investment decision to be made?	
2. Have the entrepreneurs highlighted the wants and needs that their proposed product or service will fulfill?	
3. Has the proposal clearly identified a target market for the product or service (e.g., active seniors, inactive teens, or children with a physical disability)?	
4. Has the proposal given a realistic description of the potential benefits for the intended target market?	
5. Has the proposal listed realistic potential risks (if any) to the sales of the proposed product or service?	
6. Have the entrepreneurs researched and analyzed existing competitive products or services to get a sense of the overall market?	
7. Does the pricing of the proposed product or service make sense? Would you buy it?	
8. Do the projected start-up costs of the proposed product or service make sense?	
9. Do the proposed strategies for advertising and promoting the product or service seem reasonable?	
10. Do the projected sales of the proposed product or service seem likely to make a healthy profit?	
TOTAL SCORE (out of 100)	/100

Your Investment Proposal	Presentation Points
1. Describe the features of your product or service in sufficient detail.	
2. Identify a target consumer market for the product or service (e.g., active seniors, inactive teens, or children who have a physical disability).	
3. Describe the specific wants and needs that the proposed product or service will fulfill.	
4. List the potential benefits of the product or service for the intended target market.	
5. List any potential risks that might hinder development or sales of the proposed product or service.	
6. Do some research to find out about competitive products or services to get a sense of the overall market.	
7. Establish a pricing structure for the proposed product or service that makes sense.	
8. Predict realistic start-up costs for launching the proposed product or service.	
9. Determine appropriate advertising and promotion strategies for the proposed product or service.	
10. Assess whether the projected sales of the proposed product or service will yield a profit.	

WORKSHEET

3.4 American Sport Scholarships Available to Canadians

For Canadian high school athletes, there are important issues at stake if and when they are offered a sports scholarship to the United States. The following exercise involves some research into these scholarships.

Name: _____

Date: _____

College and university sport in the U.S. is organized into Division I, Division II, and Division III and a number of regions. Two helpful websites to find out more are the official sites of the National Collegiate Athletic Association at www.ncaa.com and www.ncaa.org.

MISSION: Working in a group, choose a number of sports that interest you for which sports scholarships are available at U.S. colleges and universities. Complete the chart below by gathering information to fill in each column. A sample entry featuring the sport of women's field hockey is given below.

Sport	Number of NCAA Division One Schools That Compete in This Sport	Current NCAA Division One Championship School in This Sport (Men and Women)	A Canadian Athlete Who Competed on Scholarship (incl. Hometown and College Attended)	Number of Scholarships Available in NCAA Competition and Average $ Value
Women's Field Hockey	Total: 78	Connecticut (2014)	Maire Dineen (Toronto, ON) University of Maine	Total: 936 $14,660 per year
_____				
_____				

Sport	Number of NCAA Division One Schools That Compete in This Sport	Current NCAA Division One Championship School in This Sport (Men and Women)	A Canadian Athlete Who Competed on Scholarship (incl. Hometown and School Affiliation)	Number of Scholarships Available in NCAA Competition and Average $ Value
_____				
_____				
_____				

Chapter 3 Quiz

The two sets of questions below will test your knowledge and broaden your understanding of the material covered in Chapter 3. Complete each set of questions according to your teacher's instructions.

Name: _____

Date: _____

Question Set 1: Sport as a Business Enterprise

Multiple-Choice Questions

MISSION: Circle the letter beside the answer that you believe to be correct.

1. Amateur athletes receive compensation for their efforts through
   (a) player contracts
   (b) endorsement deals
   (c) sale of merchandise and tickets
   (d) none of the above

2. Formerly for amateurs only, the Olympic Games now permit competition by professional
   (a) skaters and ice dancers
   (b) hockey and basketball players
   (c) baseball and softball players
   (d) boxers and wrestlers

3. The largest source of profits for big-business sports teams is
   (a) athlete endorsements
   (b) ticket sales
   (c) the use of games for the sale of various rights
   (d) concession sales

4. Many sports events are broadcast as
   (a) regular over-the-air telecasts
   (b) exclusive pay-per-view engagements
   (c) live-streamed video
   (d) all of the above

5. Nike has received criticism for
   (a) the huge endorsement fees it has paid to celebrity athletes
   (b) the targeting of its marketing towards youth
   (c) the manufacturing of its products in Third World countries
   (d) its advertising at the London Olympic Games

6. Professional sports teams contribute to their local economy by
   (a) increasing sales at restaurants and hotels close to stadiums
   (b) employing people in the local community
   (c) paying taxes to the government
   (d) all of the above

Short-Answer Questions

MISSION: Briefly answer the following questions in the space provided:

1. The revenue generation associated with live sports events is similar to what other events?

2. What features are offered to viewers as part of an overall sport-as-entertainment package?

3. Which trend in athlete endorsement and marketing was ushered in by Michael Jordan's huge endorsement contract?

Essay Questions

MISSION: On a separate piece of paper, develop a 100-word response to the following questions.

1. Does a city actually benefit from hosting the Olympic Games, thereby justifying the enormous cost of preparing a bid for the IOC?

2. How do broadcasters recoup the massive sums they have paid for broadcasting rights to sporting events? What would happen if this revenue source were unavailable to them?

3. Examine arguments both for and against the role of a player's agent. Form your own opinion and provide justification for it.

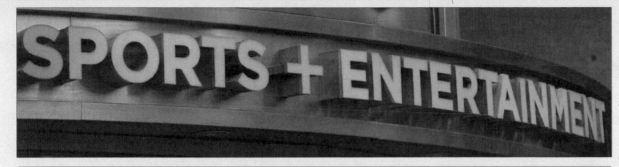

Fred Lum/The Globe and Mail

Question Set 2: Sport Media and the Sport Consumer

Multiple-Choice Questions

MISSION: Circle the letter beside the answer that you believe to be correct.

1. Technical advances in television broadcasting have led to the growth of
   (a) mobile platforms for sports events
   (b) the sport-as-entertainment industry
   (c) professional sports leagues
   (d) the fitness industry

2. The primary relationship between professional sports teams and leagues and the media is the
   (a) overall entertainment package offered to fans
   (b) viewing of games via mobile devices
   (c) blending of sports action and advertising
   (d) sales of broadcasting rights to games

3. A major threat for sports broadcasting companies is
   (a) the piracy of broadcast signals
   (b) Canada's federal Competition Bureau
   (c) increasing bandwidth fees
   (d) mergers between telecommunications giants

4. Sports fans today use social media
   (a) to receive and share scores and statistics
   (b) to follow live action or catch highlights on their computers or mobile phones
   (c) to engage in direct social exchanges with their favourite athletes
   (d) all of the above

5. We can protect ourselves from fraudulent claims made about health and wellness products by
   (a) asking friends for their opinions
   (b) buying only small samples to see if they work
   (c) relying on reliable sources of information such as Health Canada
   (d) checking out online testimonials

6. Membership contracts with pre-payment, facility-based businesses such as fitness clubs are called
   (a) renewable-option agreements
   (b) consumer alert agreements
   (c) personal development services agreements
   (d) criteria-based agreements

Short-Answer Questions

MISSION: Briefly answer the following questions in the space provided:

1. Why might it be a problem if too much sports broadcasting power is placed in the hands of just a few people?

2. What are three factors fuelling increasing sales of products and services related to health and fitness?

3. List three target markets that are especially susceptible to false or misleading advertising related to health and wellness products and services.

Essay Questions

MISSION: On a separate piece of paper, develop a 100-word response to the following questions.

1. What are the advantages and disadvantages when a company purchasing a sports team or franchise owns media outlets as well?

2. Various forms of social media have changed how fans follow sports. Are these trends positive or negative? Justify your opinion.

3. How can you become sufficiently well-informed when deciding to purchase a health product or sign up for a gym or a fitness club?

My Notes on Chapter 3

Use the space below to make notes on the questions on the facing page, to record any thoughts and ideas you have on this chapter, and to store study tips to help you prepare for tests and exams.

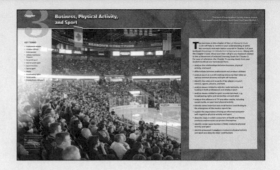

Chapter 3 Review (Student Textbook page 89)

Knowledge

1. State the differences between (a) professional athletes and amateur athletes; and (b) for-profit sport and not-for-profit sport.

2. In a graphic organizer, show all the ways in which the business world is connected to your participation in a favourite physical activity or sport.

3. How do amateur athletes qualify for funding from Sport Canada, and how much money do they typically receive per year?

4. Why are large media conglomerates such as Disney that own professional sports franchises sometimes unconcerned if their team is losing money?

5. What are the primary motivations of the key participants in the world of professional sport, i.e., owners, athletes, agents, and fans?

6. Draw a cause-and-effect map to show significant changes that have occurred in "big league" sports due to the influence of mass media.

7. Describe the relationship that is key to the huge amounts of money that change hands in the business side of professional sports, and give an example.

8. List three reasons why it is important to become an informed consumer of products and services related to physical activity and sport.

Thinking and Inquiry

9. In a table, list some pros and cons of sport spin-offs. Be as detailed as possible in your responses.

10. Nike has been criticized for producing many of its products in developing nations, thereby reducing its manufacturing costs. Examine the criticisms that Nike has faced for its "remote manufacturing" practices. Which side do you support on this issue, and why?

11. Brainstorm five athletes who are each sponsored by a major company. Why is it "good business"' for a company to sponsor an elite athlete?

12. Why do you think the Nike promotional campaign involving "regular people" during the 2012 Olympic Games was so successful?

13. Do you think that the large gaps in salaries between average players in a national sports league and the high earners in those leagues are justified? Cite specific examples in your answer.

14. In your opinion, are the huge earnings of professional athletes warranted? Justify your answer.

15. Do you think the Canadian federal government's Competition Bureau should exert stricter control over ownership deals in which a company that buys a sports team owns media outlets as well? Elaborate.

16. Analyze the relationship between business, physical activity, and sport by researching the growth of private fitness industries over the past 30 years.

17. What criteria could you use to judge whether claims made for a health and wellness product are valid?

Communication

18. As a class, debate whether professional athletes should be allowed to compete in the Olympics.

19. Select a television ad involving a top-earning professional athlete as a spokesperson, and evaluate whether the ad would be as effective if the spokesperson were a non-athlete. Explain your reasoning.

20. Prepare to evaluate and discuss the influence of the media on the world of sports. Examine the positive (+P), negative (-M), and interesting (I) influences that various media have had on the business of sport. Use a PMI chart to keep track of the class discussion.

21. If a friend were researching a fitness club to join, what three key pieces of advice would you offer?

Application

22. Based on your own experience and that of your friends, would you conclude that broadcasters and sports organizations are succeeding in attracting and retaining younger viewers as a result of social media usage? Explain your answer.

23. If you had money to invest and could start up a business to sell a product or service related to health and wellness, what type of product or service would you choose to market, and why?

24. Research a labour dispute in a professional sports league that has occurred in the last 20 years. Compare the issues underlying labour disputes researched by your classmates. As a class, make a list of recommendations for players and owners.

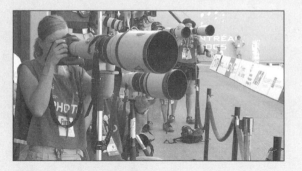

Controversy was sparked when a sports federation unanimously voted to use photographers' vests as advertising space. The photojournalists claimed that they are not "walking billboards.")CP Photo/Dimitri Papadopoulos)

Ethical Issues, Physical Activity, and Sport

KEY TERMS

- Gender-based inequities
- Canadian Association for the Advancement of Women in Sport and Physical Activity (CAAWS)
- Sport ethics
- Sport sponsorship
- Violence
- Aggression
- Cheating
- Fair play in sport
- Canadian Centre for Ethics in Sport (CCES)

From its beginnings in the late 1960s, the sport of ultimate has relied on the "spirit of the game" to maintain fair play. Players generally call their own fouls and only dispute a call when they genuinely believe a foul did not occur.

Photo by Tanya Winter

The exercises in this chapter of the *Lab Manual & Study Guide* will help to reinforce your understanding of some key concepts and main topics covered in Chapter 4 of your textbook *Kinesiology: An Introduction to Exercise Science.* Along with the Chapter 4 Quiz, these exercises will give you feedback related to the achievement of selected Learning Goals for Chapter 4. For ease of reference, the Chapter 4 Learning Goals from your student textbook are reproduced here:

- analyze the role that ethical issues play in sport at all levels

- analyze gender-based inequities in sport such as pay disparities and under-representation of women as coaches and referees

- describe efforts to overcome discrimination based on gender identity and sexual orientation in sport

- analyze the ethics of sponsorship of sporting events by manufacturers of products such as soft drinks and alcohol

- examine the prevalence of sexist and offensive advertising during televised sports events

- describe the various modes of violence and aggression that occur both on and off the sport field

- analyze serious health risks such as spinal injuries and concussions related to violence and aggression in sport

- differentiate between various ways to cheat in sport, including use of banned substances and match fixing

- compare and contrast cheating behaviours with ethical conduct that demonstrates fair play in sport

- debate whether athletes who cheat during sporting events deserve a second chance

- describe how Canadian and international organizations promote fair play ideals, such as honesty, honour, justice, inclusiveness, and drug-free sport

4.1 Gender-Based Pay Inequity in Sport

Male and female athletes today have many opportunities to experience success. However, women still face disadvantages when it comes to levels of participation, financial compensation, and endorsement deals.

Name: _____

Date: _____

MISSION: Do some research and then complete the chart below to show the differences in financial compensation in six sport leagues and events for pro male athletes versus pro female athletes.

Sport	Average Annual Salaries		Event Prize Money	
	Men	**Women**	**Men**	**Women**
Basketball	NBA $ _____	WNBA $ _____	N/A	N/A
Hockey	NHL $ _____	CWHL $ _____	N/A	N/A
Golf	N/A	N/A	Canadian Open $ _____	Canadian Pacific Women's Open $ _____
Horse racing (jockey earnings)	N/A	N/A	Queen's Plate $ _____	Queen's Plate $ _____
Nascar racing	N/A	N/A	$ _____	$ _____
Tennis (Grand Slam)	N/A	N/A	Wimbledon $ _____	Wimbledon $ _____
Tennis (Canadian)	N/A	N/A	Rogers' Cup $ _____	Rogers' Cup $ _____

MISSION: After completing your research, answer the questions below. For each question, state your opinion or make suggestions, and then provide a rationale.

1. Do you think that pay equity for male and female athletes is good for sport in general? Why or why not?

_____

_____

_____

_____

_____

_____

2. Should the media bear some responsibility to promote pay equity for men and women in professional-level sport?

_____

_____

_____

_____

_____

_____

3. What measures might (a) the Canadian federal government and (b) private corporations take to promote gender-based pay equity in Canadian sport?

_____

_____

_____

_____

_____

_____

4. Would pay equity have a positive overall impact on gender equality in a sport? Might pay equity in the world of sport have a positive influence on gender equality in society as a whole? Explain your thinking.

_____

_____

_____

_____

_____

_____

WORKSHEET

4.2 The Ethics of Sport Advertising and Sponsorships

Many unhealthy products are marketed in association with sports. For example, alcohol advertising is rampant in many sports broadcasts despite the known health risks related to excessive alcohol consumption.

Name: _____

Date: _____

Issue 1: Should Alcohol Manufacturers Be Prohibited From Sponsoring Athletes and Sports Events?

Scenario: For years, large companies all around the world have capitalized on the massive public appeal of sports in marketing a wide array of products and services. Cigarettes, alcohol, breakfast cereals, soft drinks, candy, snacks, and even "junk food" have all been endorsed by sponsors of sporting events and by high-profile athletes. These athletes receive huge financial rewards for endorsing a variety of products. However, many of these products may actually be harmful to human health. As a case in point, in Canada, cigarette companies used to sponsor tennis tournaments and curling bonspiels despite the obvious "disconnect" between smoking cigarettes and playing these sports. In 2000, however, Canadian federal laws were passed that restricted the advertisement of cigarettes at sporting events.

MISSION: Should the Canadian government ban alcohol manufacturers from sponsoring athletes and sports events? In the spaces provided below, summarize arguments for and against such a ban, and then express your own viewpoint on the issue in a well-organized paragraph.

Arguments For:

_____

_____

_____

_____

Arguments Against:

_____

_____

_____

_____

Your Viewpoint on the Issue:

_____

_____

_____

_____

_____

_____

_____

_____

Issue 2: Should Celebrity Athletes Endorse Only Healthy Food Products in Advertising Campaigns?

Scenario: In 2013, the journal *Pediatrics* published the results of an eye-opening study that found that 79 percent of 62 food products endorsed by athletes in TV, radio, and Internet advertisements were calorie-dense and nutrient-poor. About 93 percent of the 46 beverages advertised derived 100 percent of their calories from added sugar! The researchers had evaluated the nutritional quality of products endorsed by celebrities including:

- NHL player Sidney Crosby (Gatorade and Tim Hortons)
- NBA basketball superstar LeBron James (McDonald's and Sprite)
- NFL player Peyton Manning (Gatorade and Pepsi-Cola)
- Tennis player Serena Williams (Kraft Oreo cookies and Gatorade)

The study's authors proclaimed, "The promotion of energy-dense, nutrient-poor products by some of the world's most physically fit and well-known athletes is an ironic combination that sends mixed messages about diet and health." The authors also declared that "Professional athletes have an important opportunity to promote the public's health, particularly for youth, by refusing endorsement contracts" [promoting junk foods].

The authors urged governments worldwide to draw up policies that restrict advertisements of unhealthy food and beverage products featuring professional athletes in media targeted at youth.

MISSION: Complete the steps below to develop your thinking with regard to the issue of celebrity endorsements of unhealthy food products in the world of sport.

1. Find and briefly describe an example of a print, online, or TV advertisement in which an athlete endorses a product that will clearly not benefit the health and well-being of that athlete or the general public.

   _____

   _____

2. In a well-organized paragraph, explain why there is an obvious disconnect between the product and the athlete who is endorsing the product.

   _____

   _____

   _____

   _____

   _____

   _____

   _____

   _____

   _____

3. Decide whether legislation should be passed banning the endorsement of unhealthy food products by celebrity athletes. Justify your decision as persuasively as you can.

   _____

   _____

   _____

   _____

   _____

WORKSHEET

4.3 True Sport—What Constitutes "Fair Play"?

Understanding the origin of the True Sport Movement can further your appreciation of current trends and events related to ethical conduct in sport, and of how fair play principles apply in everyday situations.

Name: _____

Date: _____

Championing "Fair Play" in Sport in Canada

The concept of "fair play" is important not only in sporting situations, but in society as a whole. With this in mind, federal and provincial government leaders from across Canada met in 2001 to discuss some controversial issues that had arisen in sport.

These leaders recognized the positive impact that fair play practices in sport can have in our communities, and they sought to find a way to reduce the incidence of violence, bullying, cheating, aggressive parental behaviour, and doping in relationship to sport.

Their discussions led to the signing of the London Declaration in 2001. This Declaration was described as "an unprecedented affirmation of positive sporting values and principles."

The Canadian Centre for Ethics in Sport (CCES) then led a series of discussions across Canada to identify how to help young athletes stay on an ethical path. In the early 2000s, the CCES helped to form True Sport.

True Sport is a series of programs and initiatives that are centered upon four shared values and principles: fairness, excellence, inclusion, and fun. Schools, communities, and organizations can tap into these programs and initiatives to help promote the many positive benefits that play and sport can provide.

True Sport believes that good sport can make a profound difference in our athletes and in our communities, and thus they promote the following seven True Sport Principles.

The Seven True Sport Principles

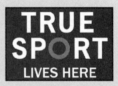

1. Keep it fun. Find the joy of sport and have a good time. Keep a positive attitude and look to make a positive difference, on the field and in your community.

2. Respect others. Show respect for everyone in creating a sporting experience, both on the field and off. Win with dignity and lose with grace.

3. Give back. Always remember the community that supports your sport and helps make it possible. Find ways to show your appreciation and help others get the most out of sport.

4. Go for it. Always strive for excellence and rise to the challenge, but never at the expense of others. Discover how good you can be.

5. Play fair. Play honestly and obey the rules in letter and spirit. Winning is only meaningful when competition is fair.

6. Stay healthy. Place physical and mental health above all other considerations and avoid unsafe activities. Respect your body and keep in shape.

7. Include everyone. Share sport with others, regardless of creed, ethnicity, gender, sexual orientation or ability. Invite everyone into sport to make it more meaningful for the whole community.

Applying the Seven True Sport Principles

MISSION: Apply the seven True Sport Principles to help you evaluate and respond to the dilemmas outlined in the scenarios below. Identify the specific True Sport Principle(s) that pertain to each scenario.

Scenario 1: You are helping out as a leader with a house league hockey team. The team is made up of boys and girls who are seven years old. You notice that the coach only chooses a few of the more talented boys to demonstrate drills. Explain how you would react to the coach's behaviour, and why.

_____

_____

_____

_____

Scenario 2: Your school's dance team has worked extremely hard over the past three years. The team members have developed outstanding skills and abilities. As a result, they have won all of the competitions they entered in the past year. If you were the coach, what more could you do to challenge your team?

_____

_____

_____

_____

Scenario 3: You are a member of your school's football team. Two students from your school have the job of holding the first-down measuring chain (which marks the distance to the first down). During a league game, you notice that the students who are holding the measuring chain have been moving the flag too far, thus giving your team an unfair advantage when you are on offence. Explain how you would react to this situation, and why.

_____

_____

_____

_____

Scenario 4: You are a pitcher for a rep softball team. You are enjoying an excellent game, pitching a no-hitter as you head towards the final inning. There are two outs and the potential last batter is at the plate. The batter connects with your pitch and sprints to first base. It appears that the runner is just barely thrown out at first, when the umpire calls her safe. Explain how you would react to the umpire's call, and why.

_____

_____

_____

_____

Scenario 5: Your friend is training hard for an upcoming track-and-field meet. She is experiencing a lot of anxiety about the outcome of the competition. She feels intense pressure to win for the glory of her team and her school, so much so that she confides to you that she is on the verge of taking a banned performance-enhancing substance. Which True Sport principle(s) would your friend violate if she resorts to using a banned performance-boosting substance? What advice would you give your friend?

_____

_____

_____

_____

WORKSHEET

Chapter 4 Quiz

The two sets of questions below will test your knowledge and broaden your understanding of the material covered in Chapter 4. Complete each set of questions according to your teacher's instructions.

Name: _____

Date: _____

Question Set 1: Sport Equity and the Ethics of Advertising and Sponsorship

Multiple-Choice Questions

MISSION: Circle the letter beside the answer that you believe to be correct.

1. Examples of gender-based inequity in sport include
   (a) prohibition of women from competing in high-profile men's professional events
   (b) lower pay for women in professional sports leagues compared to pay for men
   (c) fewer opportunities for corporate sponsorship for female athletes compared to male athletes
   (d) all of the above

2. One major sport in which men and women are compensated equally is:
   (a) basketball
   (b) race car driving
   (c) wrestling
   (d) tennis

3. According to CAAWS, gender equity in sport requires
   (a) equal access for girls and women to a full range of sport activity and program choices
   (b) identical sport programs for both sexes
   (c) "feminine" sport activity and program choices
   (d) women's participation in "male" sports

4. The first male participant in a major professional sport to come out as gay was
   (a) Mark Tewksbury
   (b) Michael Sam
   (c) Jason Collins
   (d) Greg Louganis

5. Advocates of tighter regulation of sport sponsorship by the alcohol industry liken alcohol to
   (a) cocaine
   (b) tobacco
   (c) sugar
   (d) heroin

6. The backlash against soft drink manufacturers has not been as strong as it has been against
   (a) fast food outlets
   (b) manufacturers of processed foods
   (c) manufacturers of cigarettes and alcohol
   (d) manufacturers of energy drinks

Short-Answer Questions

MISSION: Briefly answer the following questions in the space provided:

1. What is the general result of gender-based inequities in sport and in society as a whole ?

2. Who is one notable exception to the general trend of male referees officiating at men's professional sporting events?

3. Why do many observers consider gender tests administered by the IAAF to be flawed?

Essay Questions

MISSION: On a separate piece of paper, develop a 100-word response to the following questions.

1. Discuss what can be done to combat gender-based inequities in sport such as pay disparity and under-representation of women as coaches and referees.

2. Discuss ways to confront discrimination based on sexual orientation in the world of sport.

3. Analyze the prevalence of sexist and offensive advertising during televised sports events.

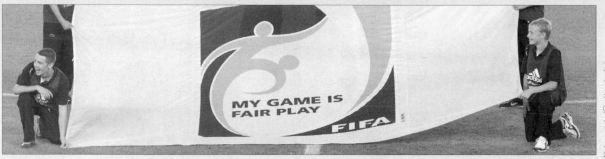

Natursports/Shutterstock

Question Set 2: Violence, Cheating, and the Fair Play Movement

Multiple-Choice Questions

MISSION: Circle the letter beside the answer that you believe to be correct.

1. Some experts claim that helmets worn by sports players cannot completely eliminate
   (a) body checking
   (b) neck injuries
   (c) spinal cord injuries
   (d) serious brain injury

2. The world soccer organization FIFA has penalized unruly soccer fans by
   (a) fining soccer teams
   (b) banning teams from competition
   (c) forcing teams to play games in empty stadiums
   (d) all of the above

3. If a serious injury prevents movements of a person's arms and legs, the injury is known as
   (a) paraplegia
   (b) quadriplegia
   (c) neuralgia
   (d) post-concussion syndrome

4. A sports player who suffers a concussion should
   (a) report it immediately to a trainer or coach
   (b) consult a doctor right away
   (c) focus on recovery so the brain has time to heal
   (d) all of the above

5. Collaboration among professional sports team owners, players, and referees to predetermine the results of a game is known as
   (a) "working the ref"
   (b) "influence peddling"
   (c) "match fixing"
   (d) "bending the rules"

6. The four core values of the True Sport Movement are
   (a) fairness, excellence, inclusion, and fun
   (b) respect, equity, dignity, and ethical conduct
   (c) friendship, team spirit, fair competition, sport without doping
   (d) tolerance, care, excellence, and the joy of movement

Short-Answer Questions

MISSION: Briefly answer the following questions in the space provided:

1. List various methods that athletes use to cheat.

2. What does it mean if a coach urges a team player to "hit hard but hit legal"?

3. Why is the role of youth-sport coaches in furthering the principles of fair play more important than ever?

Essay Questions

MISSION: On a separate piece of paper, develop a 100-word response to the following questions.

1. Discuss the issue of dangerous levels of violence and aggression in major team sports.

2. Examine the possible ethical risks if a coach promotes the attitude of "winning at all costs."

3. Explain the mandate of the Canadian Centre for Ethics in Sport.

My Notes on Chapter 4

Use the space below to make notes on the questions on the facing page, to record any thoughts and ideas you have on this chapter, and to store study tips to help you prepare for tests and exams.

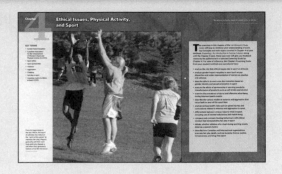

_____
_____
_____
_____
_____
_____
_____
_____
_____
_____
_____
_____
_____
_____
_____
_____
_____
_____
_____
_____
_____
_____

Chapter 4 Review (Student Textbook page 113)

Knowledge

1. How did athletes such as Kathrine Switzer help promote equal rights for women in sport and in society at large?

2. Why have many people referred to professional sport as the "last closet"?

3. Give three examples of current issues related to the ethics of sport sponsorship and advertising.

4. Identify several products that you think are unethical or questionable in relationship to endorsement by sport professionals. Explain your reasoning.

5. What forms do violence and aggression commonly take in sport today? Give some examples of the consequences of "inside-the-rules" and "outside-the-rules" violence in sport.

6. Define cheating in sport, and give examples of four different cheating behaviours on the part of athletes, coaches, and officials. What do these forms of cheating have in common?

7. With a partner, list as many values as you can related to the concept of fair play in sport, and give a real-world example of fair play in action.

Thinking and Inquiry

8. Select one example of a gender-based inequity in sport and suggest possible strategies for addressing that inequity. You may wish to do some research to support your ideas.

9. Given the humiliation experienced by South African runner Caster Semenya, do you think that major sport championships should declare themselves gender-neutral? Justify your answer as reasonably and persuasively as you can.

10. Why do you think the public backlash against sugary drink manufacturers as sports sponsors has not been nearly as strong as it has been against tobacco or alcohol manufacturers?

11. Suppose you belong to a watchdog organization that monitors sport-related sponsorship and advertising. In a group, draw up some guidelines to share with potential sponsors to ensure that their ads uphold appropriate ethical standards.

12. Describe appropriate penalties or punishment if someone intentionally injures a player, a fan, or an official during a game or competition.

13. Research an athlete who has sustained life-or career-threatening injuries during play. Some suggestions are Eric Lindros, Keith Primeau, Wade Belak, and Junior Seau. Connect what you discover about the athlete's injury to what you learned in this chapter. Present your findings in a brief report to the class.

14. "Drug use is so widespread in sports such as cycling that it is hypocritical to heap scorn only on those who are caught." Do you agree or disagree with this opinion? Give reasons for your response.

15. In June 2013, news reports revealed that the Biogenesis clinic in Miami was providing illegal steroids to at least 20 Major League Baseball players to enhance their performance. The 20 players were suspended. Research this scandal and summarize your findings.

Communication

16. Compose several questions to pose to a high-profile female coach or referee such as Violet Palmer to find out how she managed to succeed in a male-dominated field. Work with a partner research possible answers to your questions and conduct a mock radio, television, or online interview for the class.

17. Sketch a design for a billboard or a Facebook post that urges responsible drinking during sporting events.

18. Design a flyer, a poster, or a PSA (public service announcement) describing signs, symptoms, and steps to take in the event of a concussion.

19. Research an incident involving either cheating or unethical behaviour in sport or an example of exceptional good will or fair play. Create a class bulletin board display to showcase the examples.

Application

20. If you could serve as a youth advisor to an organization such as Supporting Our Youth, what strategies would you recommend to advance gender equity or respect for diverse sexual orientations?

21. Watch a sporting event on TV or online and keep a record of the commercials aired during the event. Identify (a) the target market, and (b) whether the commercial's message is healthy or unhealthy and respectful or disrespectful. Justify your responses.

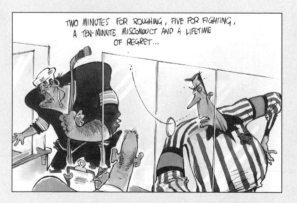

A tendency towards excessive violence on the ice has marred the careers of a number of National Hockey League players. (Editorial Cartoon by Anthony Jenkins / The Globe and Mail)

UNIT 1: SOCIETY, PHYSICAL ACTIVITY, AND SPORT

Career Choices

Investigate a career in one of the fields mentioned in this unit. Ideally, you should interview someone working within the field for this assignment. You can ask him or her the following questions and a lot more as well.

Name: _____

Date: _____

MISSION: Answer the series of questions below in relation to the career you have selected. If you interviewed a person for this career information, use quotation marks to distinguish what they said from your own comments on the career. Give the person's name and job title.

1 Career and description

_____
_____
_____
_____
_____

2 List at least two post-secondary institutions in Ontario and/or Canada that offer programs for this career.

_____
_____
_____
_____

3 Choose one of the above institutions and determine the required courses in the first year of study for this program.

_____
_____
_____
_____

4 How many years of post-secondary education are required before beginning this career? Is an internship or apprenticeship required?

_____

_____

_____

_____

5 What is the demand for individuals qualified for this occupation? If possible, provide some employment data to support your answer.

_____

_____

_____

_____

6 What is the average starting salary for this career? What is the top salary? On what do salary increases depend in this career?

_____

_____

_____

_____

7 List occupational settings where a person with these qualifications could work.

_____

_____

_____

_____

The Skeletal and Articular Systems

KEY TERMS

- Anatomical position
- Anatomical planes
- Anatomical axes
- Human skeleton
- Axial skeleton
- Appendicular skeleton
- Landmark
- Fractures
- Osteoporosis
- Articular system
- Joints
- Synovial joint
- Osteoarthritis
- Cartilage
- Dislocation
- Separation

Amy Gough starts her run during women's skeleton training at the Whistler Sliding Centre at the 2010 Olympic Winter Games in Vancouver. Amy has a passion for sports, and an athletic background as a rugby player in B.C.

CP Photo/Jeff McIntosh

"Humankind is designed for exercise and not rest—hence the legs are located below the torso. If designed for rest, we would at best have castors."

—Arthur Stewart, Scotland

The exercises in this chapter of the *Lab Manual & Study Guide* will help to reinforce your understanding of some key concepts and main topics covered in Chapter 5 of your textbook *Kinesiology: An Introduction to Exercise Science.* Along with the Chapter 5 Quiz, these exercises will give you feedback related to the achievement of selected Learning Goals for Chapter 5. For ease of reference, the Chapter 5 Learning Goals from your student textbook are reproduced here:

- use basic terminology related to anatomy and physiology

- describe the anatomical position, anatomical planes and axes, and basic movements involving joints

- describe the role and functions of the human skeleton and the skeleton's basic structure and composition (the axial skeleton and the appendicular skeleton)

- identify the five types of human bones and the names and locations of the body's key bones and bone structures

- explain the meaning of a bone "landmark"

- describe the anatomy of a long bone

- describe the main types of bone fractures and explain how bones heal

- describe the characteristics and causes of osteoarthritis and osteoporosis and the effects of aging on the skeletal system

- describe the role of joints within the human body

- describe the structural classification of joints (fibrous, cartilaginous, and synovial) and the anatomical classification of joints

- identify types and characteristics of synovial joints

- describe some common joint injuries and how to treat and prevent them

WORKSHEET

5.1 Anatomical Terminology

The "anatomical position" is the universally accepted starting point for anatomical description and analysis. Along with "planes" and "axes," this is a fundamental concept that should be grasped before moving on.

Name: _Dougie B_

Date: _Nov 22_

(A) The Anatomical Position

MISSION:

Label the visual using the labels provided below.

- ☑ **Midline**
- ☑ **Posterior/anterior**
- ☑ **Distal/proximal**
- ☑ **superior/inferior**
- ☑ **medial/lateral**

In your own words, list the main "points to remember" about the anatomical position, as described on page 118 your textbook. The main bodily orientations of the anatomical position are:

1. Anterior/Posterior = Anterior refers to [Front] of body, whereas posterior refers to back of [body]

2. Superior/Inferior = Superior refers to [upward↑] face of your body, whereas Inferior refers to [downward↓] face of body.

3. Medial/Lateral = Medial refers ← [towards] the midline of body, whereas Lateral refers to [away] of the midline.

4. Proximal/Distal = Proximal means towards the point of attachment to limb, Distal means away from limb of body.

5. midline = invisible line that goes straight down the middle of your body.

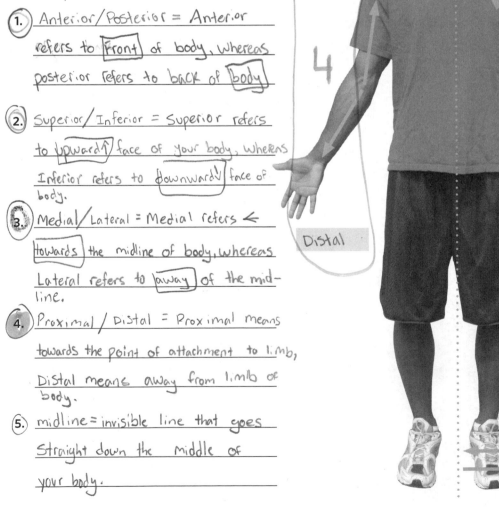

Midline
5

BACK Body
Posterior
1
front body
Anterior

Proximal

4

Superior
Face up

Distal

2
face down

Inferior

Medial

Lateral

(B) Anatomical Planes and Anatomical Axes

MISSION: Anatomical planes and anatomical axes are at right angles to each other. Label the planes and axes and then lightly colourize the planes in the illustration below. Commit them to memory to the point where you can use these terms freely to describe any movement.

☑ Antero-posterior axis
☑ Horizontal axis
☑ Longitudinal axis

☑ Sagittal plane
☑ Frontal Plane
☑ Transverse Plane

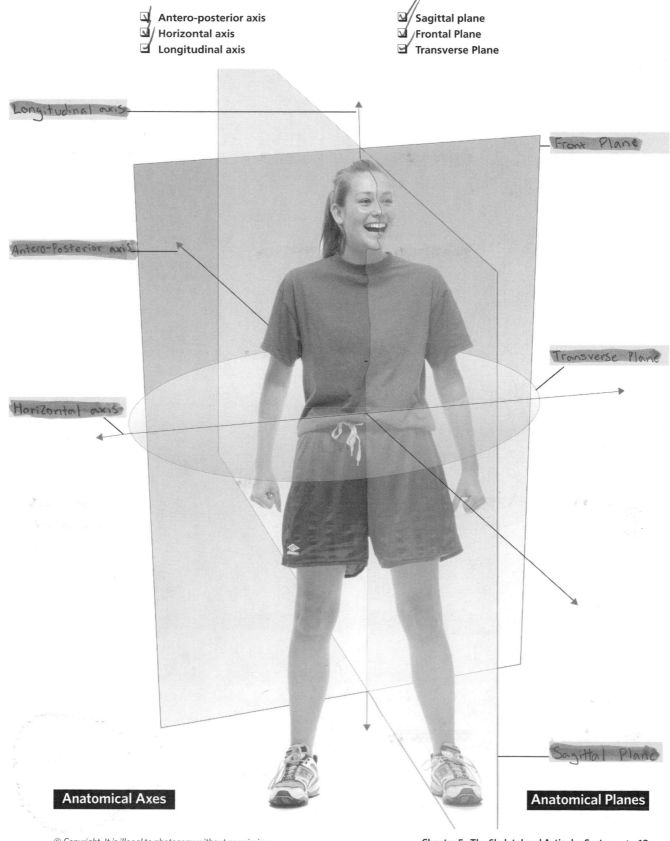

Longitudinal axis

Front Plane

Antero-Posterior axis

Transverse Plane

Horizontal axis

Sagittal Plane

Anatomical Axes

Anatomical Planes

(C) Describing Movements at Joints

Now that you have a grasp of the basic concepts (anatomical position and planes and axes), here are a few more anatomical terms that derive from these concepts and that are commonly used to describe movement.

MISSION: Label the movements below choosing the correct terms:

- ☑ Dorsiflexion / Plantar flexion
- ☑ Eversion / Inversion
- ☑ Pronation / Supination
- ☑ Flexion / Extension
- ☑ External rotation / Internal rotation
- ☑ Abduction / Adduction
- ☑ Circumduction

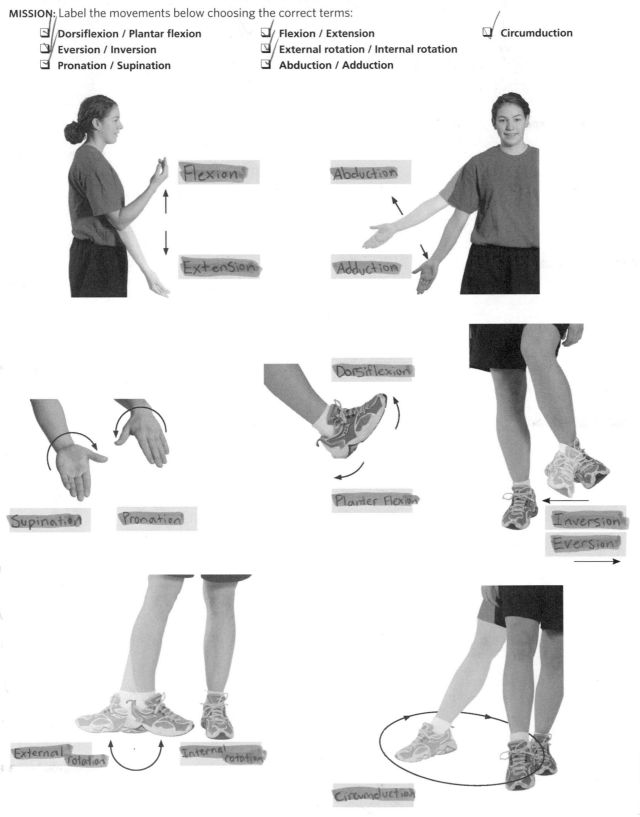

(D) Reviewing Anatomical Terminology

MISSION: Choose the correct anatomical term and write it in the second column of the chart.

Which Anatomical Term Is Correct?	
1. Straightening out your leg at the knee is an example of [**extension** / **flexion**].	Extension
2. A biceps curl is an example of arm [**flexion** / **extension**] at the elbow.	Flexion
3. Unscrewing a bottle with your right hand is in example of [**pronation** / **supination**] at the wrist.	Pronation
4. Standing on your tiptoes is an example of [**plantar flexion** / **dorsiflexion**] at the ankle.	
5. Bringing your arm in towards your sides is an example of [**adduction** / **abduction**].	adduction
6. Throwing an underhand softball pitch is an example of [**extension** / **circumduction**] at the shoulder.	Extension
7. Most common ankle injuries involved either [**eversion** / **inversion**] at the ankle joint.	Inversion
8. Shrugging to indicate a "no" response is an example of [**depression** / **elevation**] of the shoulders.	depression
9. The axis of rotation is always [**perpendicular** / **parallel**] to the plane of movement.	Perpendicular
10. The quadriceps muscles are located on the [**anterior** / **posterior**] side of the thigh.	Anterior
11. The heart is [**inferior** / **superior**] to the diaphragm muscle.	Superior
12. The elbow joint is at the [**proximal** / **distal**] end of the humerus.	Distal
13. The shoulder joint is at the [**proximal** / **distal**] end of the humerus.	Proximal
14. Tennis elbow (a tendon injury on the outer side at the elbow) involves an injury to the [**lateral** / **medial**] epicondyle.	Lateral
15. A figure skater in a spinning movement is rotating on the [**antero-posterior** / **longitudinal**] axis.	Antero posterior
16. A figure skater in a spinning movement is rotating on the [**transverse** / **sagittal**] plane.	Sagittal
17. A forward tumble by a gymnast involves rotation on the [**horizontal** / **longitudinal**] axis.	Longitudinal
18. A forward tumble by a gymnast involves rotation on the [**frontal** / **sagittal**] plane.	Frontal
19. A sideways cartwheel involves rotation on the [**antero-posterior** / **horizontal**] axis.	Antero-posterior
20. A sideways cartwheel involves rotation on the [**frontal** / **transverse**] plane.	Transverse

WORKSHEET

5.2 Major Bones in the Human Body

There are about 209 bones in the human skeleton. Many of the major ones are shown in the illustrations on these two pages.

MISSION: Find the major bones listed below. Write their name beside the correct number below.

Name: _____

Date: _____

Labels (Posterior View)

- ☑ Calcaneus
- ☑ Cervical Spine (C1–C7)
- ☐ Coccyx
- ☑ Femur
- ☑ Fibula
- ☑ Humerus
- ☐ Ilium
- ☑ Lumbar (L1–L5)
- ☐ Occipital Bone
- ☑ Parietal Bones
- ☑ Sacrum
- ☑ Sagittal Suture
- ☐ Scapula
- ☑ Thoracic Spine (T1–T12)
- ☑ Tibia

1 Sagittal Suture
2 Cervical Spine
3 Thoracic Spine
4 Lumbar
5 Sacrum
6 Parietal Bones
7 Occipital Bone
8 Scapula
9 Humerus
10 Ilium
11 Coccyx
12 Femur
13 Tibia
14 Fibula
15 Calcaneus

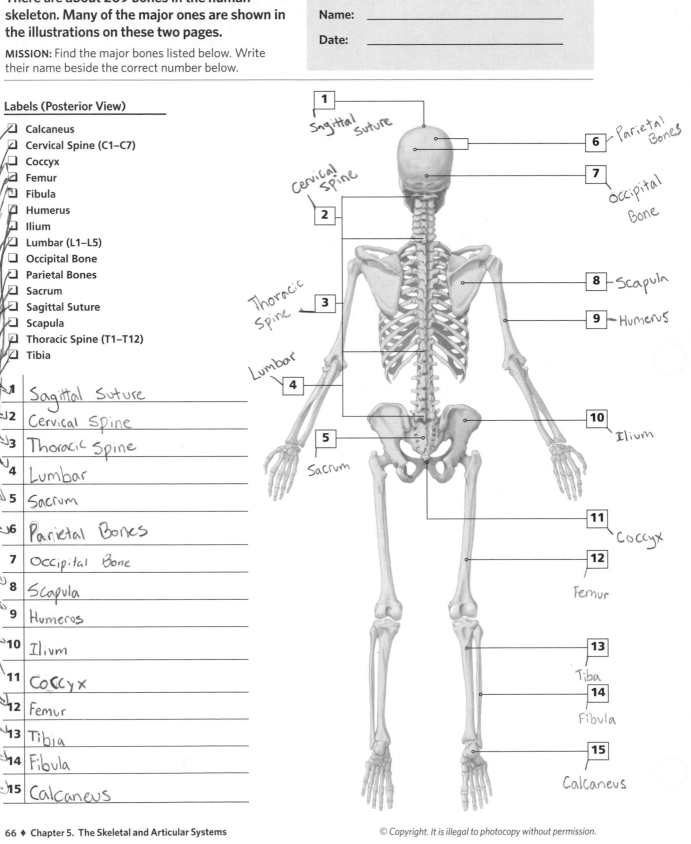

Labels (Anterior View)

- ▢ 12 Ribs
  (7 True; 3 False; 2 Floating)
- ▢ Carpals
- ▢ Clavicle
- ▢ Costal Cartilage
- ▢ Femur
- ▢ Fibula
- ▢ Frontal Bone
- ▢ Humerus

- ▢ Ilium
- ▢ Mandible
- ▢ Manubrium
- ▢ Metatarsals
- ▢ Maxilla
- ▢ Metacarpals
- ▢ Patella
- ▢ Phalanges (digits) [x 2]
- ▢ Radius

- ▢ Sacrum
- ▢ Sternum
- ▢ Symphysis Pubis
- ▢ Talus
- ▢ Temporal Bone
- ▢ Tibia
- ▢ Ulna
- ▢ Xiphoid Process
- ▢ Zygomatic Bone

#	
1	Frontal Bone
2	Temporal Bone
3	Zygomatic Bone
4	Xiphoid Process
5	12 Ribs
6	Sacrum
7	Carpals
8	Metacarpals
9	Phalanges (x1)
10	Fibula
11	Tibia
12	Maxilla
13	Mandible
14	Clavicle
15	Manubrium
16	Sternum
17	Costal Cartilage
18	Humerus
19	Radius
20	Ilium
21	Ulna
22	Symphysis Pubis
23	Femur
24	Patella
25	Talus
26	Metatarsals
27	Phalanges (x2)

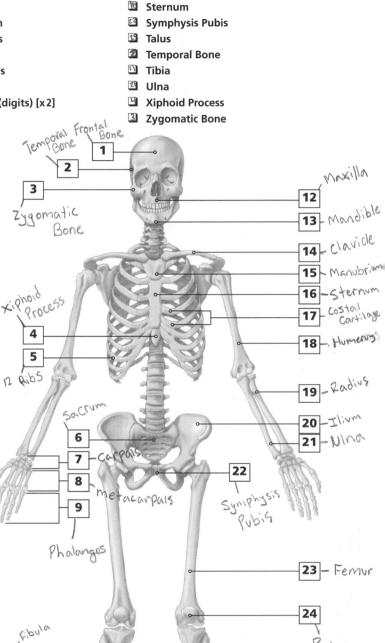

WORKSHEET

5.3 The Anatomy of a Long Bone

The long bone is the most familiar of the five basic bone types. Examples of long bones are the femur, the fibula, and the tibia.

MISSION: Label the illustration below (some labels may be used twice) using the terms on the left-hand side.

Name: _____

Date: _____

Labels

- ☑ Cartilage
- ☑ Cancellous bone
- ☐ Compact bone
- ☑ Cortex
- ☑ Diaphysis
- ☑ Epiphyseal line
- ☑ Epiphyseal plate
- ☑ Epiphysis
- ☑ Medullary cavity
- ☑ Periosteum

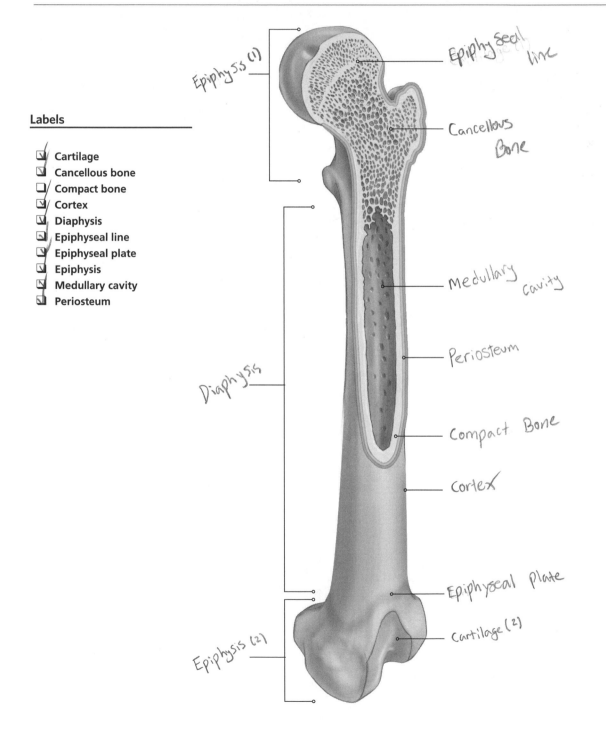

Epiphysis (1)

Epiphyseal line

Cancellous Bone

Medullary cavity

Periosteum

Compact Bone

Cortex

Diaphysis

Epiphyseal Plate

Cartilage (2)

Epiphysis (2)

WORKSHEET

5.4 Bones and Bone Landmarks

The specific locations at which major muscles, ligaments, or other connective tissue attach to bone are known as "landmarks."

MISSION: Label the illustrations on pages 69-79. Some labels may need to be used more than once.

Name: _____

Date: _____

Labels

- ☑ External auditory meatus
- ☑ Frontal bone
- ☑ Mandible
- ☐ Mastoid process
- ☑ Maxilla
- ☑ Nasal bone
- ☑ Nuchal line
- ☑ Occipital bone
- ☑ Parietal bone
- ☑ Temporal bone
- ☑ Zygomatic bone

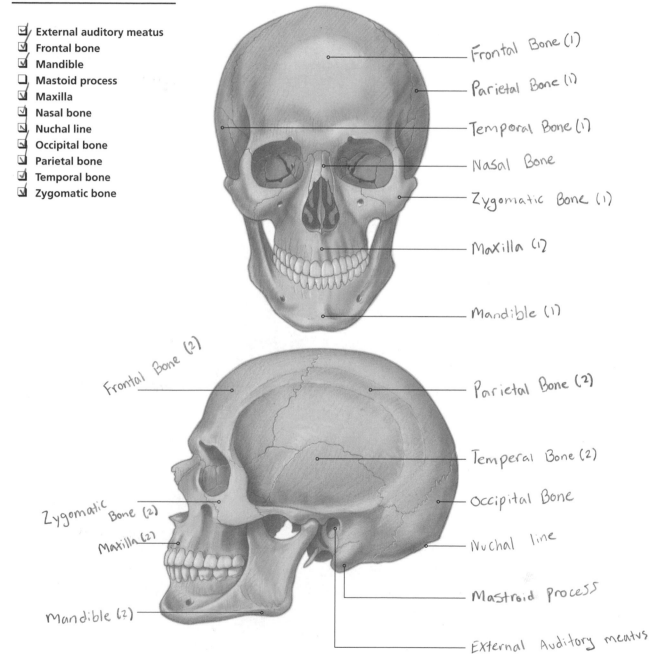

Frontal Bone (1)
Parietal Bone (1)
Temporal Bone (1)
Nasal Bone
Zygomatic Bone (1)
Maxilla (1)
Mandible (1)

Frontal Bone (2)
Parietal Bone (2)
Temperal Bone (2)
Occipital Bone
Nuchal line
Mastroid Process
External Auditory meatus
Zygomatic Bone (2)
Maxilla (2)
Mandible (2)

Labels

The vertebral column, lateral view.

- ❏ Atlas
- ❏ Axis
- ❏ Cervical region
- ❏ Coccyx
- ❏ Fifth lumbar vertebra

- ❏ First lumbar vertebra
- ❏ Intervertebral disk
- ❏ Lumbar region
- ❏ Sacral and coccygeal region
- ❏ Sacrum

- ❏ Seventh cervical vertebra
- ❏ Thoracic region
- ❏ Twelfth thoracic vertebra

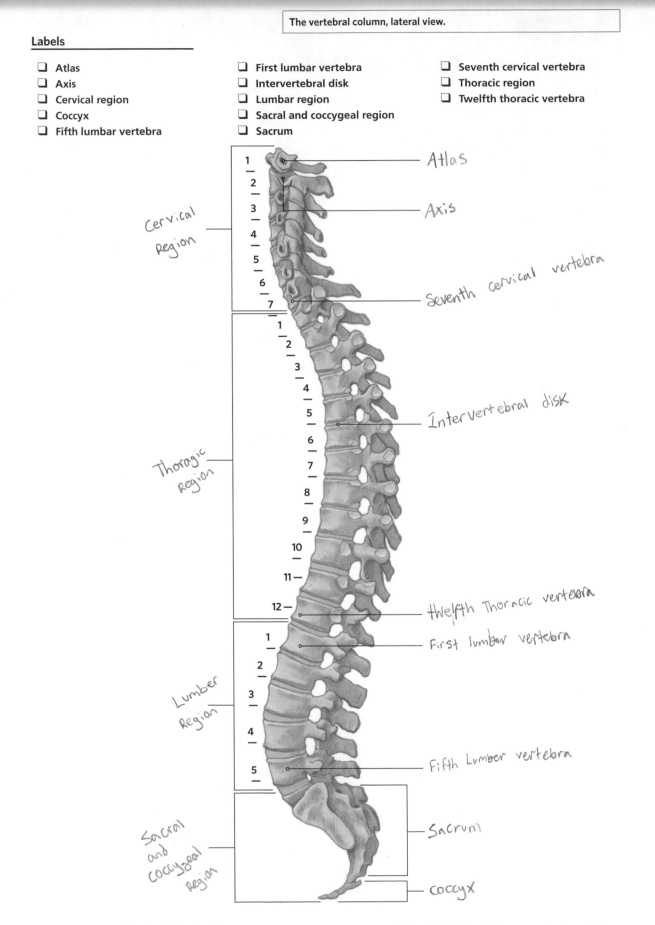

Cervical Region

Thoracic Region

Lumber Region

Sacral and coccygeal Region

1 2 3 4 5 6 7

1 2 3 4 5 6 7 8 9 10 11 12

1 2 3 4 5

Atlas

Axis

Seventh cervical vertebra

Intervertebral disk

twelfth Thoracic vertebra

First lumbar vertebra

Fifth Lumber vertebra

Sacrum

coccyx

Labels

- ☑ Body
- ☑ Clavicle
- ☑ First thoracic vertebra
- ☑ Manubrium
- ☑ Scapula
- ☑ Seven true ribs

- ☑ Sternum
- ☑ Three false ribs
- ☑ Two floating ribs
- ☑ Xiphoid process

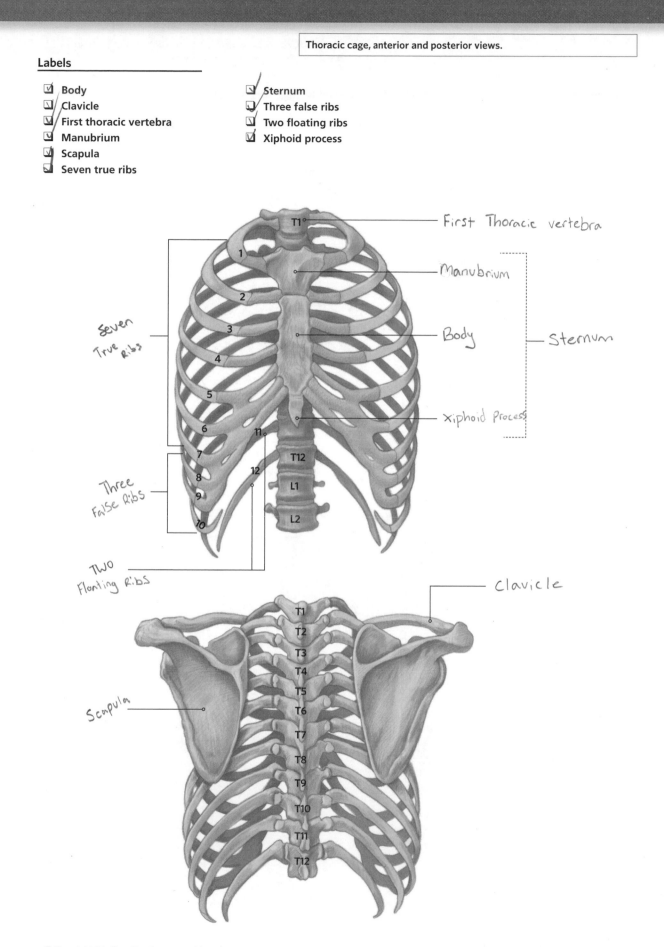

Labels

- ❑ Acromion process
- ❑ Coracoid process
- ❑ Glenoid cavity
- ❑ Glenoid fossa
- ❑ Inferior angle
- ❑ Infraglenoid tubercle

- ❑ Infraspinous fossa
- ❑ Lateral border
- ❑ Medial border
- ❑ Scapular notch
- ❑ Scapular spine
- ❑ Subscapular fossa

- ❑ Superior angle
- ❑ Supraglenoid tubercle
- ❑ Supraspinous fossa

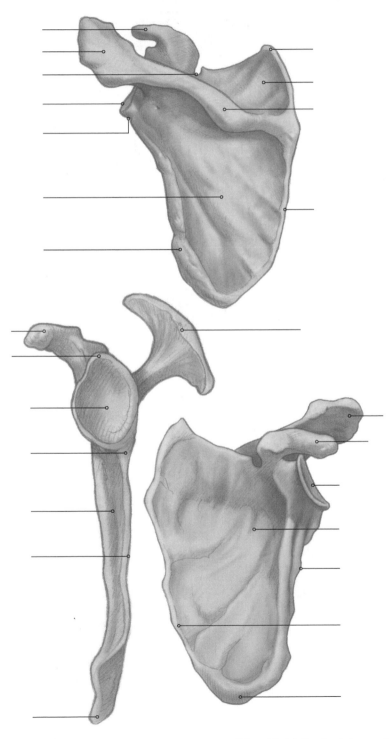

Labels

☐ Capitulum
☐ Coronoid fossa
☐ Deltoid tuberosity
☐ Greater tubercle
☐ Head

☐ Intertubercular (bicipital groove)
☐ Lateral epicondyle
☐ Lesser tubercle
☐ Medial epicondyle

☐ Olecranon fossa
☐ Radial fossa
☐ Shaft
☐ Trochlea

Left humerus, anterior and posterior views.

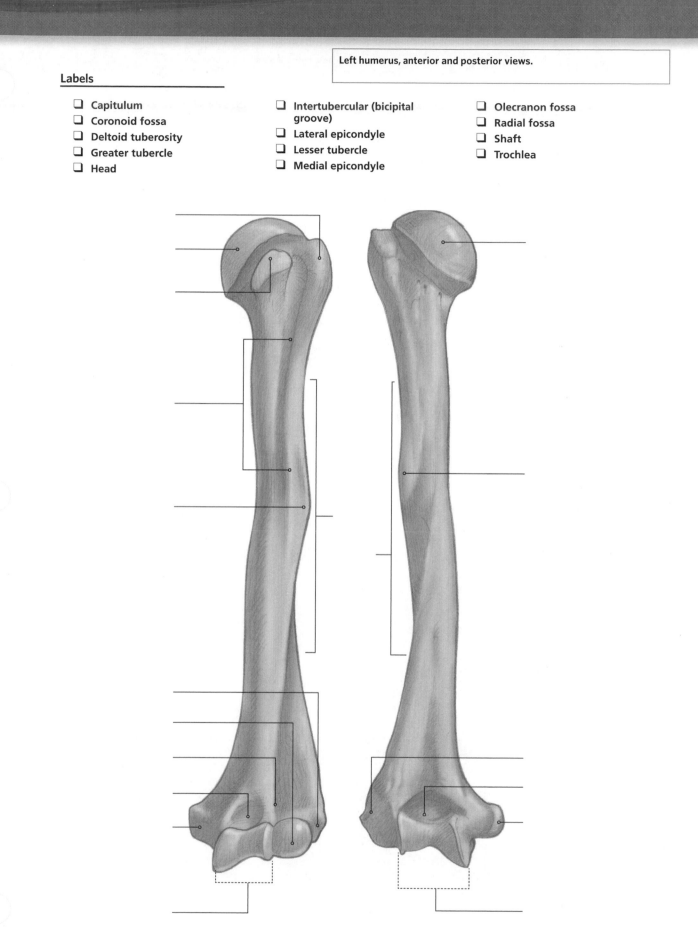

Labels

- ❏ Coronoid process
- ❏ Head
- ❏ Olecranon
- ❏ Olecranon process

- ❏ Radial notch of ulna
- ❏ Radial tuberosity
- ❏ Radius
- ❏ Styloid process of radius

- ❏ Styloid process of ulna
- ❏ Trochlear (semilunar) notch
- ❏ Ulna
- ❏ Ulna tuberosity

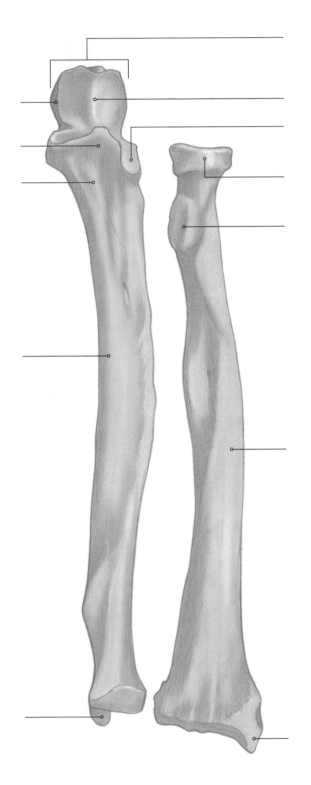

Labels

- ❏ Capitate bone
- ❏ Carpals (distal)
- ❏ Carpals (proximal)
- ❏ Distal phalanx (of finger)
- ❏ Distal phalanx (of thumb)
- ❏ Hamate bone
- ❏ Lunate bone

- ❏ Metacarpals
- ❏ Middle phalanx (of finger)
- ❏ Phalanges (Digits)
- ❏ Pisiform bone
- ❏ Proximal phalanx (of finger)
- ❏ Proximal phalanx (of thumb)
- ❏ Radius

- ❏ Scaphoid bone
- ❏ Sesamoid bone
- ❏ Trapezium bone
- ❏ Trapezoid bone
- ❏ Triquetrum bone
- ❏ Ulna

Left hand, anterior view.

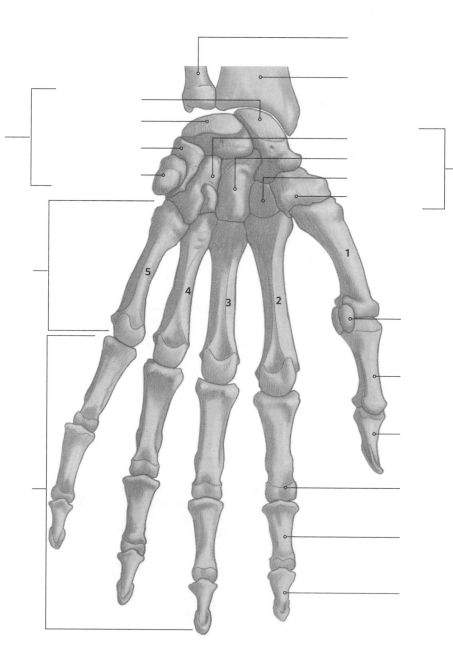

Labels

- ❑ Acetabulum
- ❑ Anterior inferior iliac spine
- ❑ Anterior superior iliac spine
- ❑ Coccyx
- ❑ Crest of ilium
- ❑ Fifth lumbar verterbra
- ❑ Ilium

- ❑ Inferior ramis of pubis
- ❑ Ischial spine
- ❑ Ischial tuberosity
- ❑ Ischium
- ❑ Obturator foramen
- ❑ Os coxae
- ❑ Posterior superior iliac spine

- ❑ Pubis
- ❑ Sacroiliac joint
- ❑ Sacrum
- ❑ Superior ramis of pubis
- ❑ Symphysis pubis
- ❑ Posterior inferior iliac spine

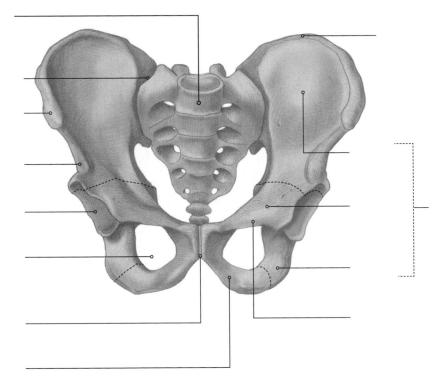

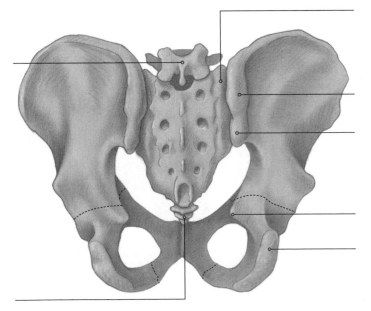

Labels

- [ ] Adductor tubercle
- [ ] Gluteal tuberosity
- [ ] Greater trochanter
- [ ] Head
- [ ] Intercondylar fossa
- [ ] Intertrochanteric crest

- [ ] Intertrochanteric line
- [ ] Lateral condyle
- [ ] Lateral epicondyle
- [ ] Lesser trochanter
- [ ] Linea aspera
- [ ] Medial condyle

- [ ] Medial epicondyle
- [ ] Neck
- [ ] Patellar groove
- [ ] Pectineal line
- [ ] Shaft

Right femur, anterior and posterior views.

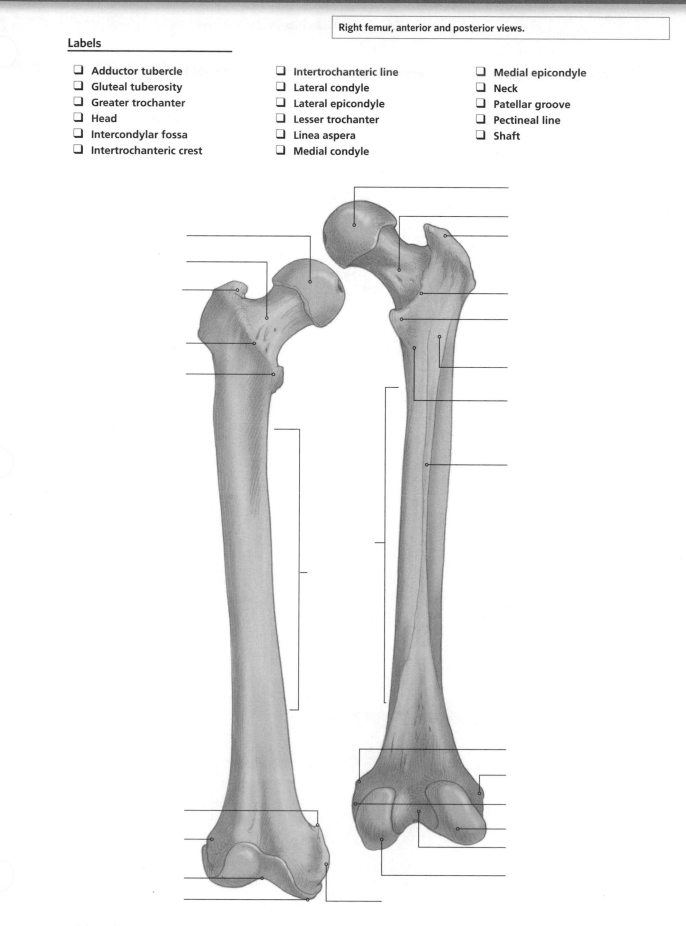

Labels

- ❏ Anterior crest
- ❏ Fibula
- ❏ Head
- ❏ Intercondylar eminence

- ❏ Lateral condyle
- ❏ Lateral condyle of tibia
- ❏ Lateral malleolus
- ❏ Medial condyle

- ❏ Medial condyle of tibia
- ❏ Medial malleolus
- ❏ Tibia
- ❏ Tibial tuberosity

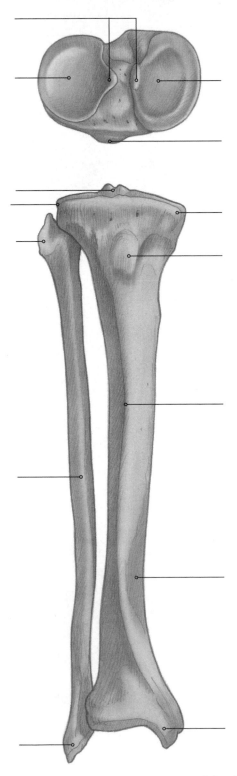

Labels

- ❑ Calcaneus
- ❑ Cuboid
- ❑ Distal phalanx
- ❑ Distal phalanx (of great toe)
- ❑ Intermediate cuneiform
- ❑ Lateral cuneiform
- ❑ Medial cuneiform
- ❑ Metatarsals
- ❑ Middle phalanx
- ❑ Navicular
- ❑ Phalanges (Digits)
- ❑ Promixal phalanx
- ❑ Proximal phalanx (of great toe)
- ❑ Talus
- ❑ Tarsals

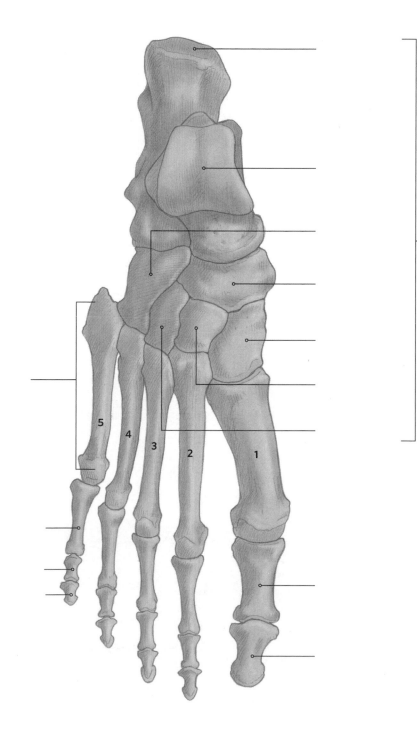

WORKSHEET

5.5 Bone Landmarks—Review Exercise

A bone "landmark" refers to a feature on a bone—a ridge, bump, groove, depression, or prominence. Landmarks are the specific locations at which major muscles, ligaments, or other connective tissue attach to bone.

Name: _____

Date: _____

MISSION: Review the illustrations on pages 69-79 and locate the landmarks listed below. Place a check mark in the box once you have found each landmark, and colour-code the box as well as the area of the bone.

Bone	Important Landmarks
Skull	☐ mastoid process
	☐ nuchal line
Vertebral column	☐ cervical
	☐ thoracic
	☐ lumbar
Sternum	☐ manubrium
	☐ body
	☐ xiphoid process
Clavicle	☐ body
Rib cage	☐ ribs 1–12
Scapula	☐ coracoid process
	☐ acromion process
	☐ supraglenoid tubercle
	☐ infraglenoid tubercle
	☐ spine of scapula
	☐ lateral border
	☐ inferior angle
	☐ superior angle
	☐ medial border
	☐ supraspinous fossa
	☐ infraspinous fossa
	☐ subscapular fossa

Bone	Important Landmarks
Humerus	☐ greater tubercle
	☐ lesser tubercle
	☐ intertubercular groove
	☐ deltoid tuberosity
	☐ surface
	☐ medial epicondyle
	☐ lateral epicondyle
Radius	☐ radial tuberosity
	☐ styloid process
	☐ surface
Wrist and hand	☐ surface
	☐ metacarpals
Ulna	☐ surface
	☐ olecranon
	☐ coronoid process
Pelvic girdle	☐ iliac crest
	☐ sacrum
	☐ anterior superior iliac spine
	☐ anterior inferior iliac spine
	☐ pubic crest
	☐ pubis
	☐ ilium
	☐ ischial tuberosity
Femur	☐ surface
	☐ greater trochanter
	☐ lesser trochanter
	☐ medial condyle
	☐ lateral condyle
	☐ adductor tubercle
	☐ linea aspera
Tibia	☐ surface
	☐ medial condyle
	☐ lateral condyle
	☐ tibial tuberosity
Fibula	☐ body
	☐ head
Calcaneus/tarsals	☐ posterior side

5.6 The Characteristics of a Synovial Joint

Synovial joints are one of the three major types of joints in the human body. They permit movement between two or more bones.

MISSION: To gain familiarity with the main aspects of the synovial joint, label the illustration below.

Name: _____

Date: _____

Labels

- ❏ Articular cartilage
- ❏ Blood vessel
- ❏ Bone

- ❏ Bursa
- ❏ Joint capsule
- ❏ Joint cavity
  (filled with synovial fluid)

- ❏ Nerve
- ❏ Synovial membrane
- ❏ Tendon

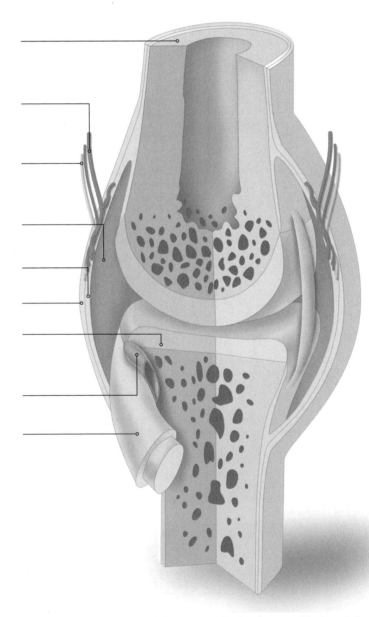

WORKSHEET

5.7 Constructing a Model of a Synovial Joint

Synovial joints are comprised of: cartilage, the joint capsule, synovia, the joint cavity, the bursae, and ligaments (intrinsic and extrinsic).

MISSION: List the components needed to construct a movable joint (the joint must be able to articulate).

Name: _____

Date: _____

Name(s) of team members	
Name of joint (your choice)	
Due date and timelines	
Research sources (e.g., Internet, visit physiotherapy clinic, etc.)	

Materials Required to Construct the Joint

Bones and joints (e.g., wooden dowels; paper towel rolls; tennis balls; hinges; pipes; plumbing couplings)	
Cartilage (e.g., concave plastic from a water bottle; modelling clay; plasticene)	
Ligaments (e.g., Velcro; pipe cleaners; plastic ties)	
Tendons (e.g., rubber bands; wire; string)	
Muscles (e.g., partially inflated balloons filled with flour)	

5.8 The Shoulder and Knee Joints

Because of their size and composition, the shoulders and knees are key joints in the human body. They are complex structures. This exercise will help you understand how they help us move about.

Name: _____

Date: _____

MISSION: Label the main components of the shoulder joint illustrated below, as well as the four anatomical views of the knee joint on the following pages. Some labels may need to be used more than once.

Labels

- ❑ Acromioclavicular ligament
- ❑ Acromion
- ❑ Clavicle
- ❑ Coracoacromial ligament

- ❑ Coracoclavicular ligament
- ❑ Coracoid process
- ❑ Glenohumeral ligaments and joint capsule

- ❑ Humerus
- ❑ Scapula
- ❑ Tendon of biceps brachii (long head)

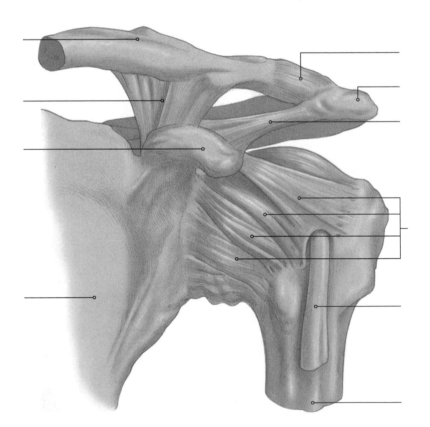

Left shoulder joint, anterior view.

Labels

- Anterior cruciate ligament
- Femur
- Fibula
- Lateral (Fibular) collateral ligament removed
- Lateral condyle
- Lateral meniscus

- Medial condyle
- Medial (Tibial) collateral ligament
- Medial (Tibial) collateral ligament removed
- Medial meniscus
- Patella (wrapped within a tendon—sesamoid bone)

- Patellar ligament
- Posterior cruciate ligament
- Quadriceps tendon (patellar tendon)
- Tibia
- Tibial tuberosity

Labels

- Adductor magnus tendon
- Anterior cruciate ligament
- Femur
- Fibula
- Fibular head
- Lateral (Fibular) collateral ligament

- Lateral head of gastrocnemius tendon
- Lateral meniscus
- Medial (Tibial) collateral ligament
- Medial head of gastrocnemius tendon
- Medial meniscus

- Oblique popliteal ligament
- Popliteal tendon
- Posterior cruciate ligament
- Posterior meniscofemoral ligament
- Semimembranosus tendon
- Tibia

5.9 Describing Movements at Joints

Joints and the surrounding muscles can be strengthened using different types of exercises. You may wish to complete this exercise after you have learned about the human muscular system in Chapter 6.

Name: _____

Date: _____

MISSION: In the worksheet below, indicate which are the main muscles in use, the joints involved, and the type of movement that is produced. A sample entry is provided below.

Exercises	Major Muscles	Joints Involved	Movement Produced
Bench press	pectoralis major, anterior deltoid, and triceps brachii	elbow and shoulder	elbow extension and medial shoulder rotation and flexion
Dumbbell flies			
Front lat pull-downs (not behind head)			
Shoulder press			
Leg curls			
Squats			
Front plank			
Shoulder shrug			
Triceps extension			
Push-ups			
McGill crunches			
Power clean			
Arm curls			

Chapter 5 Quiz

The two sets of questions below will test your knowledge and broaden your understanding of the material covered in Chapter 5. Complete each set of questions according to your teacher's instructions.

Name: _____

Date: _____

Question Set 1: Anatomical Terminology and the Human Skeletal System

Multiple-Choice Questions

MISSION: Circle the letter beside the answer that you believe to be correct.

1. The standard starting point for human anatomical description and analysis is
   (a) the axial and appendicular skeleton
   (b) anatomical planes and axes
   (c) the anatomical position
   (d) the long bone

2. As opposed to the axial skeleton, the appendicular skeleton
   (a) is the division of the skeleton from which all muscles originate
   (b) features the sternum as its central aspect
   (c) can only be seen from the anterior view
   (d) includes the limbs and plays a key role in allowing us to move

3. The nutrients and blood in bones are found in the
   (a) periosteum
   (b) diaphysis
   (c) articulating cartilage
   (d) bone marrow

4. Tendons usually unite and attach to the
   (a) periosteum
   (b) diaphysis
   (c) articulating cartilage
   (d) bone marrow

5. The structure found on the ends of long bones is the
   (a) periosteum
   (b) diaphysis
   (c) articulating cartilage
   (d) bone marrow

6. Bones attach to other bones across joints by means of
   (a) tendons
   (b) cartilage
   (c) ligaments
   (d) muscle

Short-Answer Questions

MISSION: Briefly answer the following questions in the space provided:

1. List the five main functions of the skeletal system.

2. Name the five types of bones and give an example of each type.

3. What is meant by a bone "landmark"?

Essay Questions

MISSION: On a separate piece of paper, develop a 100-word response to the following questions.

1. Long bones play a major role in our bodily movements. Sketch and describe the main components and features of a long bone.

2. What are some habits and behaviours that can help us to maintain and strengthen our skeletal system as we age?

3. What is the difference between osteoarthritis and osteoporosis? Who is particularly vulnerable to the condition known as osteoporosis? Explain why.

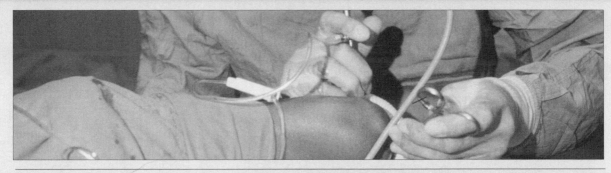

CP Photo/Phototake

Question Set 2: Joints and Joint-Related Injuries

Multiple-Choice Questions

MISSION: Circle the letter beside the answer that you believe to be correct.

1. Which of the following best describes a synovial joint?
   (a) articulating cartilage located on the ends of the bones that come in contact protects them
   (b) features a joint cavity filled with synovial fluid
   (c) permits movement between two or more bones
   (d) all of the above

2. Which of the following synovial joints is a ball-and-socket joint?
   (a) knee joint
   (b) metatarsal joints
   (c) hip joint
   (d) radioulnar joint

3. Which of the following joints is classified as uni-axial?
   (a) shoulder joint
   (b) elbow joint
   (c) carpal joints
   (d) thumb joint

4. Thick bands of fibrous connective tissue that help reinforce the joint and joint capsule are called
   (a) bursae
   (b) ligaments
   (c) tendons
   (d) cartilage

5. Which of the following bone(s) make up the shoulder joint?
   (a) clavicle
   (b) scapula
   (c) humerus
   (d) all of the above

6. Which of the following muscles help to stabilize the knee joint on the anterior side?
   (a) hamstrings
   (b) quadriceps
   (c) gastrocnemius
   (d) gluteus maximus

Short-Answer Questions

MISSION: Briefly answer the following questions in the space provided:

1. Joints are classified by structure and by function. Name the three types of joints, giving an example of each type.

2. The synovial joint is the most common joint in the human body, What are the six different types of synovial joints?

3. Distinguish the difference between first-, second-, and third-degree tears, sprains, and pulls.

Essay Questions

MISSION: On a separate piece of paper, develop a 100-word response to the following questions.

1. The synovial joint is the type of joint closely associated with human movement. Sketch and describe its main features.

2. List at least five common joint-related injuries and describe the proper treatment for an injury to a joint.

3. Summarize which type of activities or sports tend to cause injury to the shoulder and ankle joints, and explain the nature of these injuries and why they occur frequently.

WORKSHEET

My Notes on Chapter 5

Use the space below to make notes on the questions on the facing page, to record any thoughts and ideas you have on this chapter, and to store study tips to help you prepare for tests and exams.

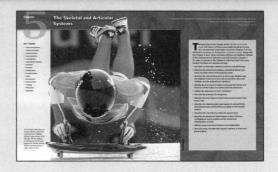

Chapter 5 Review (Student Textbook page 161)

Knowledge

1. Define the anatomical position.

2. In terms of the anatomical position, state the opposite of each of the following terms: (a) anterior, (b) superior, (c) medial, (d) proximal, and (e) superficial. Then define each pair of terms that physiologists use in relation to the anatomical position.

3. Describe the structure and functions of the two major divisions of the human skeleton and give three examples of bones in each division.

4. Name the five types of bones found in the human body and give one example of each type.

5. Name and describe the three main types of joints in the human body, based on structural classification. Give an example of each type of joint. Which type of joint allows the most human movement?

6. List the six main types of synovial joints in the human body and give an example of each type.

7. Match the shoulder joint, knee joint, and ankle joint to each of its structural and anatomical classifications as well as to the types of movement each joint permits.

8. Identify and describe major types and causes of injuries affecting (a) the shoulder joint, (b) the knee joint, and (c) the ankle joint. Which ligaments are commonly involved in these injuries? What kinds of movements or actions can lead to these injuries?

Thinking and Inquiry

9. Differentiate between the three anatomical planes and the three anatomical axes of the human body.

10. Human bones are often presented as if they were dead body tissue, but they are actually composed of living tissue. Explain how this misconception might have developed.

11. Osteoporosis is a bone disease. Osteoarthritis is a disease of the joints. Compare and contrast these two diseases with respect to causes, symptoms, and treatment.

12. Analyze how the six main characteristics of the synovial joint enable continuous, heavy use of this type of joint over many years.

13. What advice could you give (a) professional athletes and (b) everyday athletes to help them avoid joint injuries while performing or working out?

14. Athletes who use their arms to throw a ball or swing a racquet are particularly vulnerable to rotator cuff tears. Identify the damage sustained when this type of joint injury occurs, and outline some possible strategies that might help athletes reduce the risks of experiencing a rotator cuff tear.

Communication

15. State the general rule pertaining to the relationship of anatomical axes and anatomical planes to one another. Then draw simple labelled sketches showing an example of a body movement involving each combination of plane and axis.

16. Using an actual human bone or a model or illustration of one, make a presentation to your class to demonstrate the anatomy of a long bone.

17. Cartilage damage, sprains, dislocations, and separations are common joint injuries. Design a table to compare and contrast these injuries in terms of causes, signs or symptoms, and treatment.

18. In groups of three, with each person in a group assigned one joint, take turns explaining the structure and function of the shoulder joint, knee joint, and ankle joint. First, write out your description in a paragraph or two and then, one by one, read your description to your group. Describe the joint and how it works in your own words as concisely as possible.

Application

19. Using your own body (starting from the anatomical position), name and demonstrate each of the 19 types of movement that can occur at joints.

20. Work in groups of five or six, with each person responsible for a major bone in the human body (his or her choice). Taking turns, each student will present a mini-lesson to the group about the categorization and characteristics of that particular bone.

21. Based on your participation in your favourite physical activities or sports, to which joint injuries or diseases would you predict you might be most vulnerable, and why? What precautions can you take to avoid these injuries?

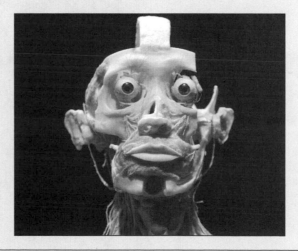

A specially preserved human head is displayed during the opening of the exhibition "Koerperwelten" (Body Worlds) staged by German professor of anatomy, Dr. Gunther von Hagens, in Heidelberg, Germany, in 2009. (AP Photo/Daniel Roland)

The Muscular System

KEY TERMS

- Musculoskeletal system
- Agonist and antagonist muscle pairs
- Origin and insertion
- Skeletal muscle fibre
- Sarcolemma
- Sarcoplasm
- Sarcomere
- Sarcoplasmic reticulum
- Neuromuscular system
- Neuromuscular junction
- Motor unit
- All-or-none principle
- Delayed onset muscle soreness (DOMS)
- Tendonitis
- Sliding filament theory
- Adenosine triphosphate (ATP)
- Reflex arc
- Proprioceptors
- Muscle spindles
- Golgi tendon organs

The Rugby Gladiators, 2007, part of the "Body Worlds and the Mirror of Time" exhibition in London, England, in 2008. Scientist and educator Dr. Gunther von Hagens' art shows the form, beauty, function, and potential of the human body.

CP Photo /Nils Jorgensen/Rex Features

The exercises in this chapter of the *Lab Manual & Study Guide* will help to reinforce your understanding of some key concepts and main topics covered in Chapter 6 of your textbook *Kinesiology: An Introduction to Exercise Science.* Along with the Chapter 6 Quiz, these exercises will give you feedback related to the achievement of selected Learning Goals for Chapter 6. For ease of reference, the Chapter 6 Learning Goals from your student textbook are reproduced here:

- identify three types of muscles (cardiac, smooth, and skeletal) and their unique roles in the muscular system

- describe the major components and primary functions of the musculoskeletal (locomotor) system and how this system allows us to move

- differentiate between agonist and antagonist muscles

- identify the major muscles and muscle groups in the human body, their location throughout the human body, and their origin, insertion, and function

- describe the anatomy of skeletal muscle

- describe the neuromuscular system and the relationship between the muscles and the nervous system

- explain the motor unit, the concept of muscle twitch, and the all-or-none principle

- identify common muscle and tendon injuries and how to treat them

- explain the contraction of muscles, the three basic kinds of contraction, the sliding filament theory of muscle contraction, and excitation-contraction coupling

- explain proprioception and the control of movement

- demonstrate an understanding of the sequence of nerve impulses and motions involved in the stretch reflex

WORKSHEET

6.1   Major Muscles of the Human Body

Skeletal muscles are those that are attached to bones (by tendons and other tissues). They are the most prevalent type of muscle in the human body, comprising 30 to 40 percent of a person's body weight.

Name: Dougie B

Date:

MISSION: Label the illustrations on these two pages using the labels provided at the top of the facing page.

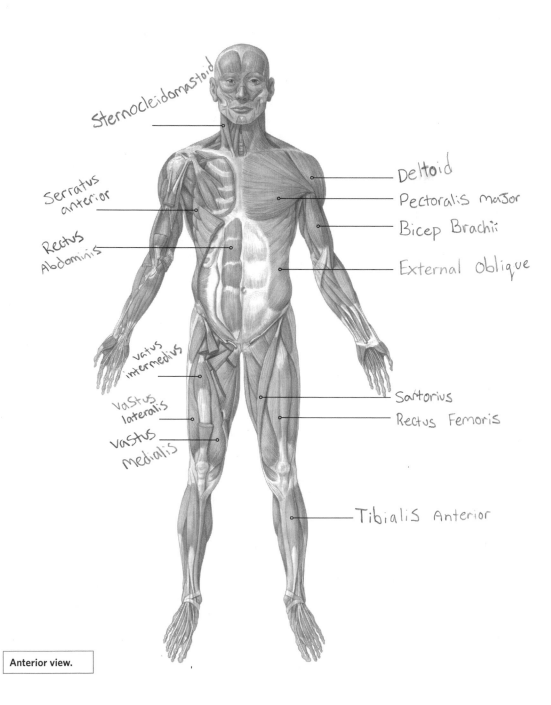

Sternocleidomastoid

Serratus anterior

Rectus Abdominis

vatus intermedius

Vastus lateralis

Vastus medialis

Deltoid

Pectoralis major

Bicep Brachii

External Oblique

Sartorius

Rectus Femoris

Tibialis Anterior

Anterior view.

☑	Biceps Brachii	☑	Pectoralis Major	☑	Sternocleidomastoid
☑	Biceps Femoris	☑	Rectus Abdominis	☐	Supraspinatus
☑	Deltoid	☑	Rectus Femoris	☑	Teres Minor
☑	External Oblique	☑	Rhomboid Major	☑	Tibialis Anterior
☑	Gastrocnemius	☑	Sartorius	☑	Trapezius
☑	Gluteus Medius	☑	Semimembranosus	☑	Triceps Brachii
☑	Gluteus Maximus	☑	Semitendonosis	☑	Vastus Intermedius
☑	Infraspinatus	☑	Serratus Anterior	☑	Vastus Lateralis
☑	Latissimus Dorsi	☑	Soleus	☑	Vastus Medialis

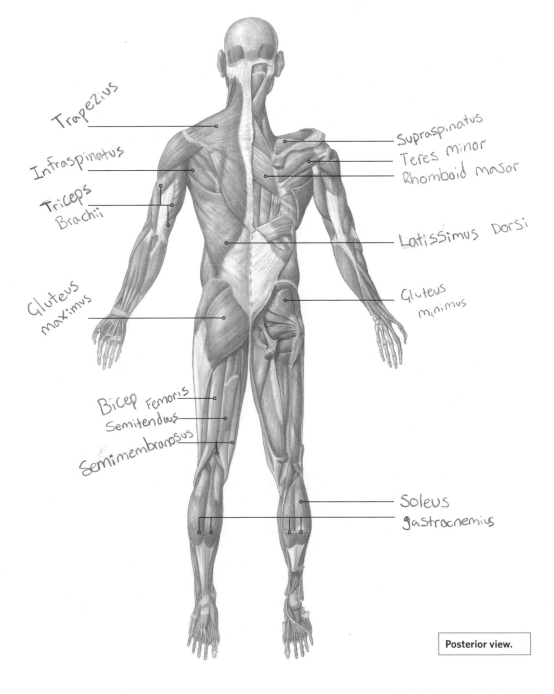

Trapezius

Infraspinatus

Triceps Brachii

Gluteus maximus

Bicep Femoris

Semitendous

Semimembranosus

Supraspinatus

Teres minor

Rhomboid major

Latissimus Dorsi

Gluteus minimus

Soleus

gastrocnemius

Posterior view.

MISSION: Using highlighters or pencil crayons, highlight the muscle names in the table on the right, and then use the same colour to shade in the muscle in the illustrations below.

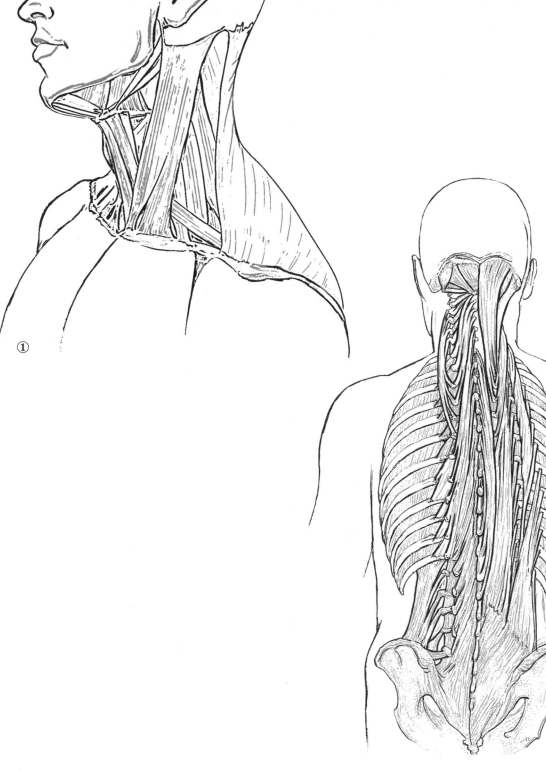

①

②

WORKSHEET

6.2 Origin, Insertion, and Function

The point where a muscle attaches to the more stationary of the bones of the axial skeleton is known as the origin. The other end, the point where the muscle attaches to the bone that is moved most, is known as the insertion.

Name: _____

Date: _____

MISSION: For the exercises on pages 96-113, complete the following tasks: (1) fill in the chart by providng each muscle's origin, insertion, and function; (2) label the illustrations on the adjacent page; (3) colour-code each muscle name in the chart so that it corresponds with the muscle in the illustration.

Exercise 6.2(a): Muscles of the Neck and Vertebral Column			
	Origin	Insertion	Function
Muscles of the Neck			
☐ STERNO-CLEIDOMASTOID			
☐ SPLENIUS			
☐ SCALENUS ANTERIOR			
☐ SCALENUS MEDIUS			
☐ SEMISPINALIS CAPITIS			
Deep Muscles of the Vertebral Column			
☐ SPINALIS			
☐ LONGISSIMUS			
☐ ILIOCOSTALIS			

Top: Muscles of the anterior thoracic wall, (1) posterior view.

Bottom: Muscles of the abdominal wall, (2) lateral superficial view.

MISSION: Using highlighters or pencil crayons, highlight the muscle names in the table on the right, and then use the same colour to shade in the muscle in the illustrations below.

①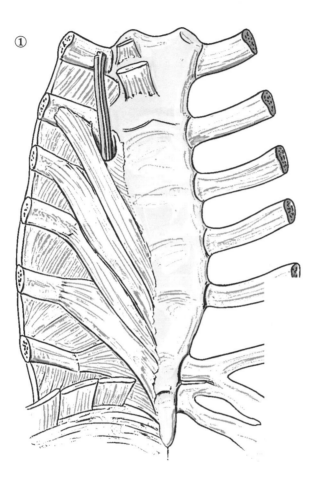

②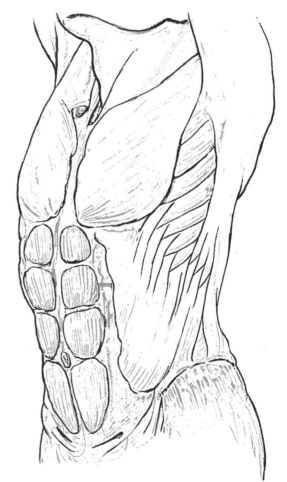

Exercise 6.2(b): Muscles of Respiration and the Abdomen

The muscles of the thoracic cage are mainly involved with breathing; those of the abdominal wall, with flexion and rotation of the vertebral column. When included with the back muscles, these groups represent the major muscles of the trunk.

	Origin	Insertion	Function
Muscles of the Thoracic Cage			
☐ THE DIAPHRAGM			
☐ INTERCOSTAL MUSCLES			
☐ TRANSVERSUS THORACIS			
Muscles of the Abdomen			
☐ RECTUS ABDOMINIS			
☐ EXTERNAL OBLIQUE AND TRANSVERSUS ABDOMINIS			
☐ QUADRATUS LUMBORUM			

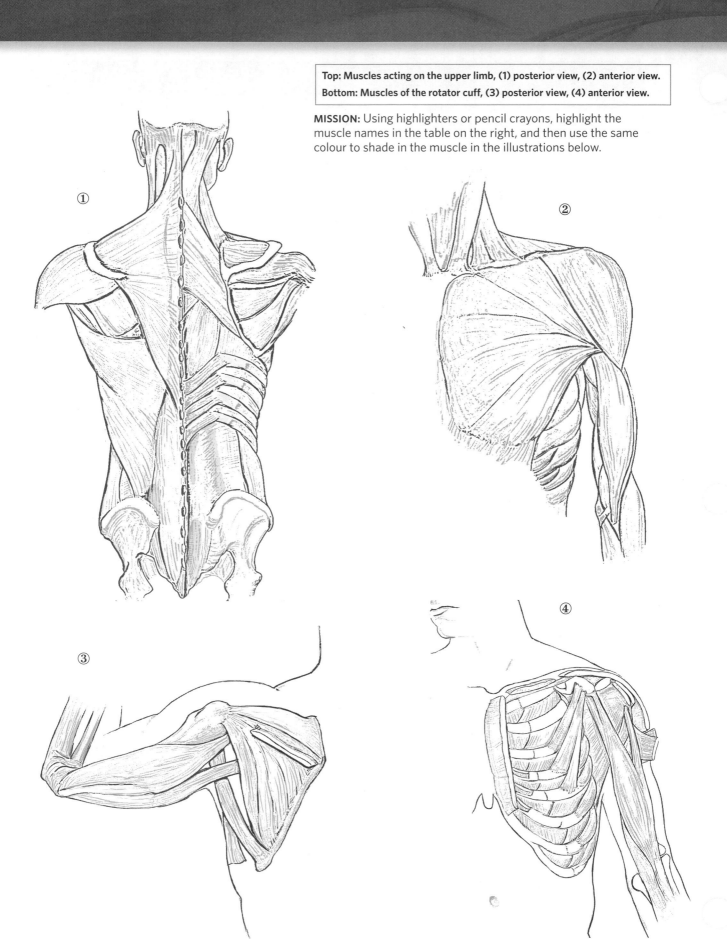

Top: Muscles acting on the upper limb, (1) posterior view, (2) anterior view.
Bottom: Muscles of the rotator cuff, (3) posterior view, (4) anterior view.

MISSION: Using highlighters or pencil crayons, highlight the muscle names in the table on the right, and then use the same colour to shade in the muscle in the illustrations below.

① ② ③ ④

Exercise 6.2(c): Muscles of the Shoulder

The muscles that affect the shoulder joint can be grouped into four categories. Two large muscles serve mainly to act on the upper limb of the axial skeleton, and four rotator cuff muscles act directly to stabilize and rotate the joint itself. The other two sets of shoulder muscles (those more directly associated with the scapula) are considered in the following section.

	Origin	Insertion	Function

Muscles Acting on the Upper Limb

These superficial muscles act on the upper limb.

	Origin	Insertion	Function
☐ PECTORALIS MAJOR			
☐ LATISSIMUS DORSI			

Muscles of the Rotator Cuff

The rotator cuff (musculotendinous cuff) consists of four muscles that extend from the scapula to the humerus and wrap around the shoulder joint, essentially holding it in place. The group is commonly referred to as the S.I.T.S. or S.S.I.T. muscles (an acronym of the muscle names) because they "sit" on the shoulder girdle. In addition to stabilizing the shoulder joint, the rotator cuff helps to decelerate arm movements (e.g., during a throwing action). If any of the rotator cuff muscles is damaged, due to strain or bad mechanics, the consequences are serious for actions that involve the shoulder and arm.

☐ SUPRA-SPINATUS			
☐ INFRA-SPINATUS			
☐ TERES MINOR			
☐ SUB-SCAPULARIS			

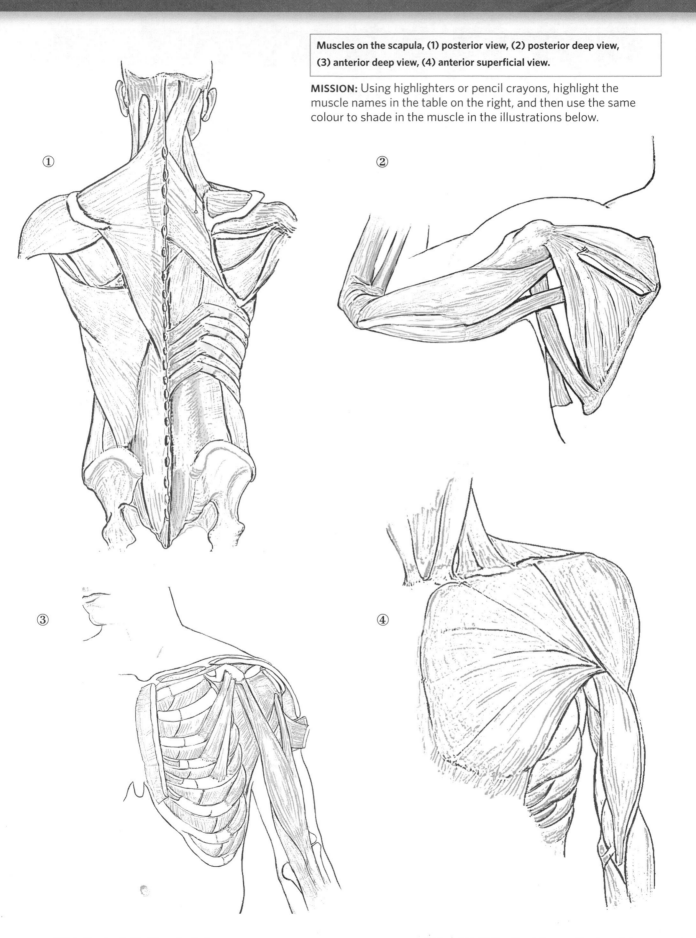

Muscles on the scapula, (1) posterior view, (2) posterior deep view,
(3) anterior deep view, (4) anterior superficial view.

MISSION: Using highlighters or pencil crayons, highlight the
muscle names in the table on the right, and then use the same
colour to shade in the muscle in the illustrations below.

Exercise 6.2(d): Muscles that Act on the Scapula

The scapula facilitates a wide range of movement at the shoulder. Apart from the rotator cuff muscles, the scapular muscles can be grouped into two categories: (1) those anchoring it to the axial skeleton, and (2) those muscles directly acting on the humerus.

	Origin	Insertion	Function
Muscles that Position the Scapula			
☐ TRAPEZIUS			
☐ RHOMBOID MAJOR AND MINOR			
☐ LEVATOR SCAPULAE			
☐ SERRATUS ANTERIOR			
☐ PECTORALIS MINOR			
Scapular Muscles that Move the Humerus			
☐ DELTOID			
☐ CORACO-BRACHIALIS			
☐ TERES MAJOR			

MISSION: Using highlighters or pencil crayons, highlight the muscle names in the table on the right, and then use the same colour to shade in the muscle in the illustrations below.

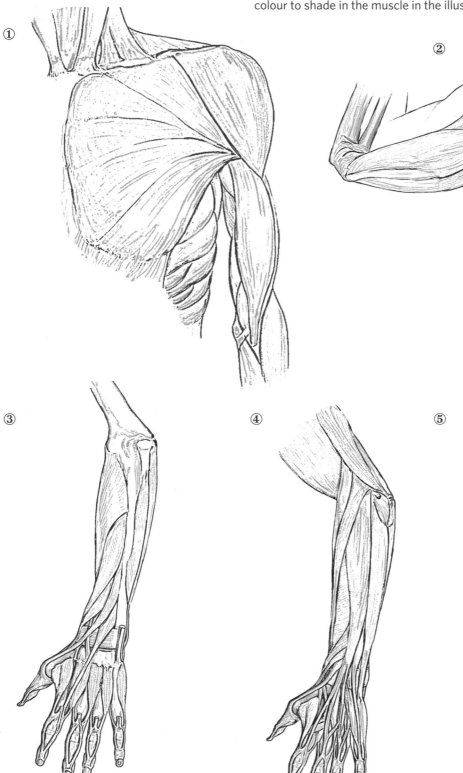

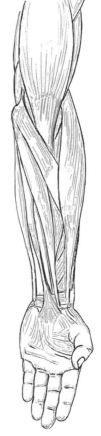

① ② ③ ④ ⑤

Exercise 6.2(e): Muscles of the Arm

The muscles of the arm control the movement of the forearm. Two major groups can be distinguished — those muscles that flex and extend the elbow (the elbow flexors and extensors) and those responsible for pronation and supination of the forearm.

	Origin	Insertion	Function
Elbow Flexors and Extensors			
☐ BICEPS BRACHII ("BICEPS")			
☐ BRACHIALIS			
☐ TRICEPS BRACHII			
☐ BRACHIO-RADIALIS			
☐ ANCONEUS			
Supination and Pronation of the Forearm			
☐ PRONATOR QUADRATUS			
☐ PRONATOR TERES			
☐ SUPINATOR			

Top: Extrinsic hand muscles, (1) anterior view, (2) posterior view.

Bottom: Intrinsic hand muscles, (3) anterior view.

MISSION: Using highlighters or pencil crayons, highlight the muscle names in the table on the right, and then use the same colour to shade in the muscle in the illustrations below.

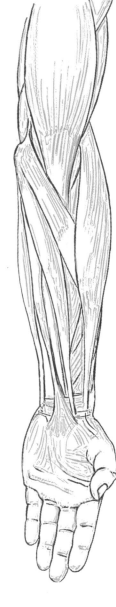

① ② ③

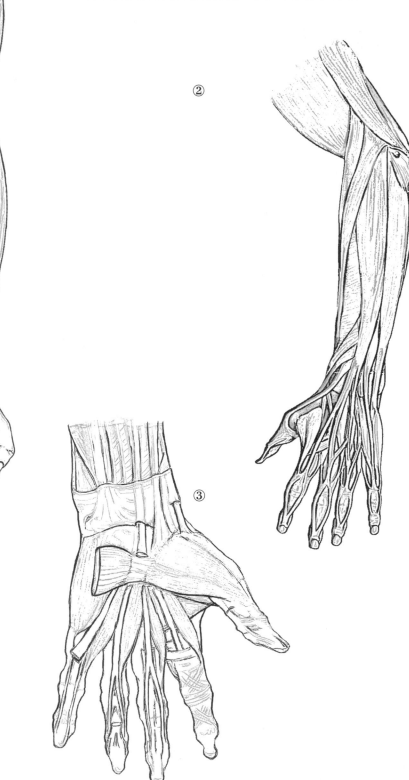

Exercise 6.2(f): Muscles of the Forearm and Hand

The muscles of the forearm (extrinsic hand muscles) are responsible for flexion, extension, abduction, and adduction of the wrist. The intrinsic hand muscles are those contained within the hand itself.

	Origin	Insertion	Function
Extrinsic Hand Muscles			
☐ FLEXOR CARPI RADIALIS			
☐ PALMARIS LONGUS			
☐ FLEXOR CARPI ULNARIS			
☐ FLEXOR DIGITORUM SUPERFICIALIS			
☐ EXTENSOR CARPI RADIALIS LONGUS			
☐ EXTENSOR CARPI RADIALIS BREVIS			
☐ EXTENSOR CARPI ULNARIS			
☐ EXTENSOR DIGITORUM			
☐ EXTENSOR DIGIT MINIMI			
Intrinsic Hand Muscles			
☐ THENAR EMINENCE			
☐ HYPOTHENAR EMINENCE			

MISSION: Using highlighters or pencil crayons, highlight the muscle names in the table on the right, and then use the same colour to shade in the muscle in the illustrations below.

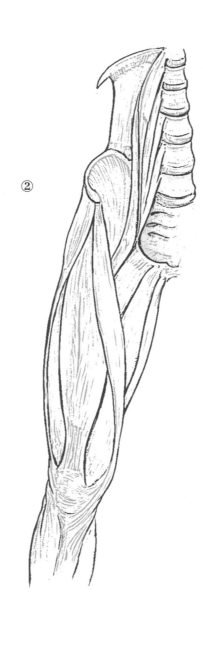

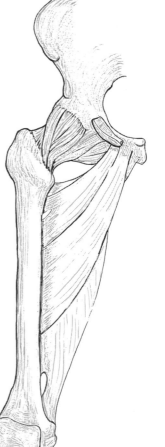

Exercise 6.2(g): Muscles of the Hip			
	Origin	Insertion	Function
Posterior Hip Muscles			
☐ GLUTEUS MAXIMUS			
☐ GLUTEUS MEDIUS			
☐ GLUTEUS MINIMUS			
☐ TENSOR FASCIAE LATAE			
☐ SARTORIUS			
Anterior Hip Muscles			
☐ ILIOPSOAS			
☐ PSOAS MINOR			
Hip Adductors			
☐ ADDUCTOR LONGUS			
☐ ADDUCTOR MAGNUS			
☐ ADDUCTOR BREVIS			
☐ PECTINEUS			
☐ GRACILIS			

Quadriceps and hamstring muscle groups, (1) anterior view, (2) posterior view.

MISSION: Using highlighters or pencil crayons, highlight the muscle names in the table on the right, and then use the same colour to shade in the muscle in the illustrations below.

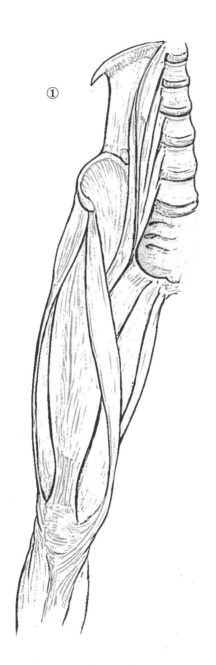

①

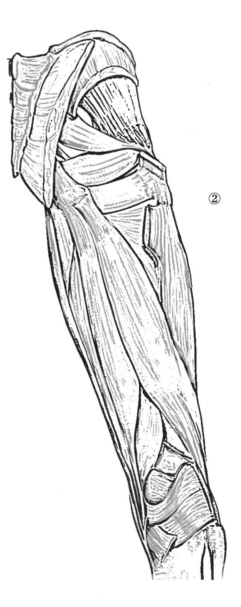

②

Exercise 6.2 (h): Muscles of the Thigh			
	Origin	Insertion	Function

Anterior Thigh—Quadriceps Group

The muscles of the anterior thigh include the quadriceps femoris group. Quadriceps femoris is the large muscle group that covers the front and sides of the thigh. In this group, there are four separate muscles (hence the "quad"): rectus femoris, vastus lateralis, vastus medialis, and vastus intermedius.

	Origin	Insertion	Function
☐ RECTUS FEMORIS			
☐ VASTUS LATERALIS			
☐ VASTUS INTERMEDIUS			
☐ VASTUS MEDIALIS			

Posterior Thigh—Hamstring Group

There are three muscles of the posterior thigh. They are referred to collectively as "the hamstrings." These muscles are: the biceps femoris, the semimembranosus, and the semitendinosus.

	Origin	Insertion	Function
☐ BICEPS FEMORIS			
☐ SEMI-MEMBRANOSUS			
☐ SEMI-TENDINOSUS			

Extrinsic foot muscles, (1) posterior deeper view, (2) anterior view, (3) posterior deep view. Intrinsic foot muscles, plantar views, (4) superficial, (5) deep, (6) intermediate.

MISSION: Using highlighters or pencil crayons, highlight the muscle names in the table on the right, and then use the same colour to shade in the muscle in the illustrations below.

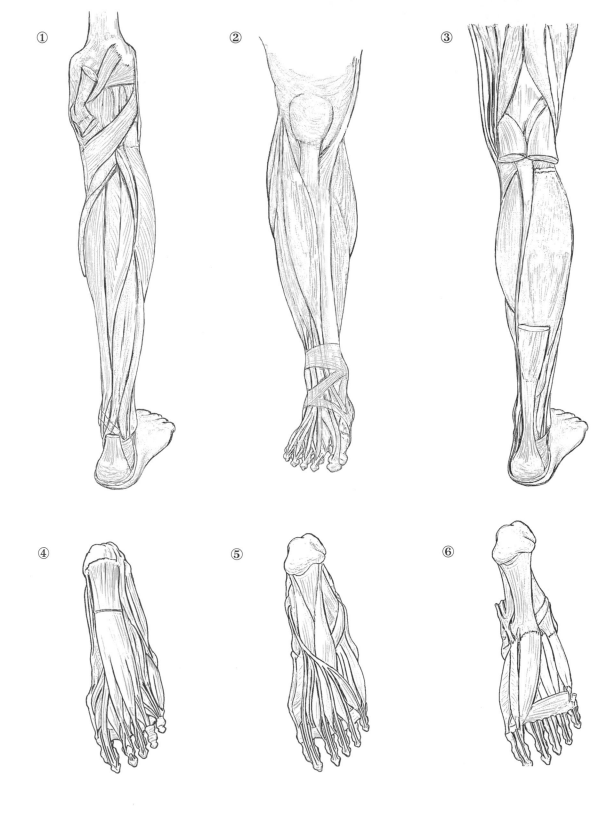

Exercise 6.2(i): Muscles of the Leg and Foot

Anatomically speaking, the "leg" refers to the lower limb below the knee. The muscles of the leg can be categorized into two broad groups, the extrinsic foot muscles and the intrinsic foot muscles.

	Origin	Insertion	Function
Extrinsic Foot Muscles			
☐ EXTENSOR DIGITORUM LONGUS			
☐ EXTENSOR HALLUCIS LONGUS			
☐ TIBIALIS ANTERIOR			
☐ GASTROCNEMIUS			
☐ SOLEUS			
☐ FLEXOR DIGITORUM LONGUS			
☐ FLEXOR HALLUCIS LONGUS			
☐ TIBIALIS POSTERIOR			
☐ POPLITEUS			
☐ FIBULARIS BREVIS & FIBULARIS LONGUS			
Intrinsic Foot Muscles			
☐ FLEXOR DIGITORUM BREVIS			
☐ QUADRATUS PLANTAE			
☐ FLEXOR HALLUCIS BREVIS			

Anterior (rows: Extensor Digitorum Longus, Extensor Hallucis Longus, Tibialis Anterior)

Posterior (rows: Gastrocnemius, Soleus, Flexor Digitorum Longus, Flexor Hallucis Longus, Tibialis Posterior, Popliteus)

Lateral (row: Fibularis Brevis & Fibularis Longus)

6.3 Agonist and Antagonist Muscle Pairs

In a muscle pair, the agonist muscle is primarily responsible for the movement of a body part (bone), whereas the antagonist muscle counteracts and lengthens when the agonist muscle contracts.

Name: _____

Date: _____

MISSION: Indicate the opposing muscle or muscle group in the table below.

Agonist	Antagonist
Triceps	
Pectoralis major	
Hamstrings	
Trapezius	
Gluteus maximus	
Erector spinae group	
Gastrocnemius	
Wrist flexors	
Supinator	
Tibialis anterior	
Anterior deltoid	
Latissimus dorsi	
Iliacus	
Adductor magnus	
External obliques	
Infraspinatus	
Rhomboids	
Sternocleidomastoid	

WORKSHEET

6.4 The Anatomy of Skeletal Muscle

The basic unit of skeletal muscle is the individual skeletal muscle fibre or muscle cell. Looking outward and inward from this basic unit shows how skeletal muscle as a whole is constructed and how it functions.

Name: _____

Date: _____

MISSION: To gain familiarity with how skeletal muscle is constructed, label the key parts of the muscle and muscle fibre in the diagrams below. Some labels may need to be used more than once.

Labels

- ☐ Tendon
- ☐ Perimysium
- ☐ Epimysium
- ☐ Endomysium
- ☐ Sarcomere (partially contracted)
- ☐ Actin

- ☐ Muscle fibre
- ☐ Myofibril
- ☐ Myosin
- ☐ Sarcolemma (muscle membrane)
- ☐ Sarcoplasmic reticulum (web-like)
- ☐ Z-line

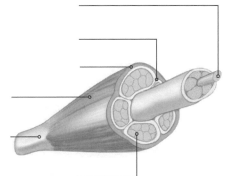
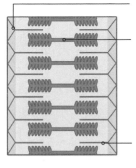

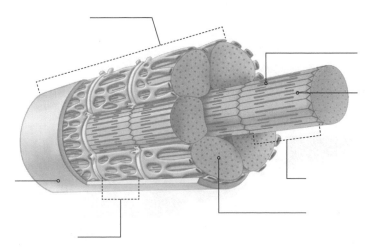

The structure of skeletal muscle.

6.5 The Neuromuscular System

The neuromuscular system is a general term referring to the complex linkage between the muscular system and the nervous system. It includes the brain, the spinal cord, the muscle fibres, and the neurons connecting them.

Name: _____

Date: _____

MISSION: To gain familiarity with the components of the neuromuscular system and neuromuscular junction, label the illustrations below.

Labels

- ❏ Axon
- ❏ Axon terminal
- ❏ Motor neuron
- ❏ Muscle fibres
- ❏ Neurotransmitter acetylcholine (ACh)
- ❏ Receptor
- ❏ Sarcolemma
- ❏ Synaptic cleft

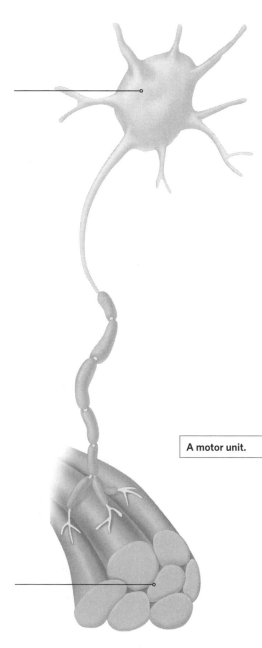

A motor unit.

A neuromuscular junction.

WORKSHEET

6.6 Excitation-Contraction Coupling

Muscles work by converting chemical energy (ATP) into mechanical energy, but muscle contraction starts with an electrical impulse from the central nervous system. This process is known as "excitation-contraction coupling."

Name: _____

Date: _____

MISSION: A sequence of events occurs before, during, and after muscle contraction—for example, when you abduct your arm. The steps are described below. The initial, middle, and final steps are numbered correctly below. Re-number the other steps in the process in the correct order of their occurrence.

1	**A message originates and is released from the central nervous system.**
	ACh causes the sarcoplasmic reticulum to release calcium ions from the terminal cisterna.
	The message is carried through the axon terminal via acetylcholine (ACh) to the sarcolemma of each muscle fibre involved.
	The message then travels from the axon branch to the axon terminal of the deltoid muscle. Since the weight is minimal, only a few muscle fibres (a small motor unit) will be recruited.
5	**The calcium ions then find their way to attachment sites on troponin, which are located on the actin's tropomyosin.**
	The myosin heads attach themselves to the binding sites on actin.
	ATP is broken down by ATPase, causing the power stroke and the sliding of actin along the myosin filament.
	The tropomyosin swivels, causing the binding sites for myosin on the actin filament to be exposed.
9	**Contraction of the filaments will continue until you decide to stop the activation of the deltoid muscle. As long as calcium is present, contraction will continue.**

6.7 The Reflex Arc

Reflex actions are how the body responds rapidly to painful—or the threat of painful—situations. The reflex arc is the pathway along which an initial stimulus and a corresponding response message travel.

Name: _____

Date: _____

MISSION: Label the illustration below using the labels on the left, and briefly describe the five components of the reflex arc in the space provided below.

1. _____

2. _____

3. _____

4. _____

5. _____

Labels

- ❑ Effector Organ
- ❑ Interneuron
- ❑ Motor Neuron (efferent)
- ❑ Sensory Receptor
- ❑ Sensory Neuron (afferent)

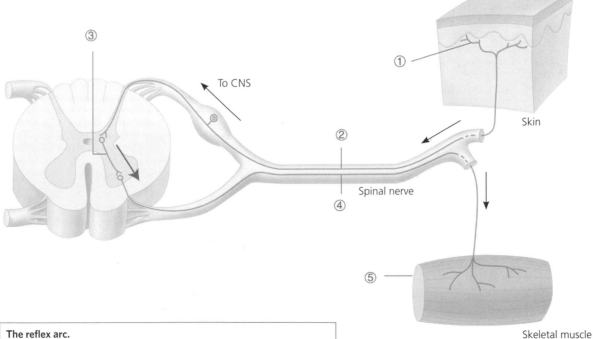

The reflex arc.

WORKSHEET

6.8 Golgi Tendon Organs at Work

Golgi tendon organs are highly specialized proprioceptors (sensory receptors) found at the end of muscle fibres that merge into the tendon itself and that detect changes in muscle tension on the tendon.

Name: _____

Date: _____

MISSION: The illustration below shows a tension reflex action involving the Golgi tendon organs. Referring to the components already labelled in the illustration below, list and describe the various stages of this reflex action.

1. _____

2. _____

3. _____

4. _____

5. _____

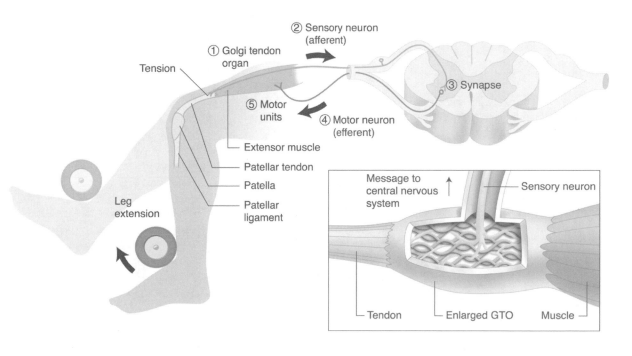

Golgi tendon organ (tension detector).

Chapter 6 Quiz

The two sets of questions below will test your knowledge and broaden your understanding of the material covered in Chapter 6. Complete each set of questions according to your teacher's instructions.

Name: _____

Date: _____

Question Set 1: The Musculoskeletal and Neuromuscular Systems

Multiple-Choice Questions

MISSION: Circle the letter beside the answer that you believe to be correct.

1. The type of muscle associated with voluntary movement is referred to as
   (a) cardiac muscle
   (b) smooth muscle
   (c) skeletal muscle
   (d) none of the above

2. Skeletal muscle attaches to bone by means of
   (a) ligaments
   (b) cartilage
   (c) muscle fibre
   (d) tendons

3. Which of the following muscles dorsiflexes the ankle?
   (a) gastrocnemius
   (b) soleus
   (c) gluteus maximus
   (d) tibialis anterior

4. Which of the following muscles flex the knee?
   (a) semitendinosus, semimembranosus, and rectus femoris
   (b) vastus lateralis, vastus intermedius, vastus medialis, and rectus femoris
   (c) supraspinatus, infraspinatus, teres minor, and subscapularis
   (d) none of the above

5. Which muscles insert on the tibial tuberosity?
   (a) semitendinosus, semifemoris, and biceps femoris
   (b) vastus lateralis, vastus medialis, vastus intermedius, and rectus femoris
   (c) semitendinosus and biceps femoris
   (d) gracilis, pectineus, and adductor brevis

6. Which muscles make up the rotator cuff?
   (a) trapezius, deltoid, and latissimus dorsi
   (b) biceps brachii, triceps brachii
   (c) supraspinatus, infraspinatus, teres minor, and subscapularis
   (d) iliopsoas, psoas major, and biceps brachii

Short-Answer Questions

MISSION: Briefly answer the following questions in the space provided:

1. What is meant by "agonist and antagonist muscle pairs"? Give an example.

2. List and describe the five properties of skeletal muscle that play a role in how muscles are named.

3. What is meant by muscle "origin and insertion"?

Essay Questions

MISSION: On a separate piece of paper, develop a 100-word response to the following questions.

1. Describe how the neuromuscular junction functions as a critical part of the neuromuscular system. You may use a sketch in your answer.

2. Explain how motor units function according to a rule known as the "all or none principle" in relation to muscle contraction.

3. What are the most common muscle and tendon injuries and in what general ways are they treated?

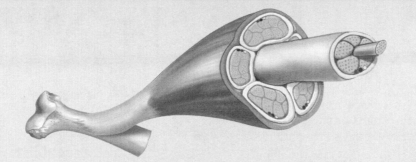

Question Set 2: The Sliding Filament Theory, Proprioception, and the Body's Reflexes

Multiple-Choice Questions

MISSION: Circle the letter beside the answer that you believe to be correct.

1. On a molecular level, during a muscle contraction, which structures attach, rotate, detach, and reattach in rapid succession in a ratchet-like fashion?
   (a) thick filaments
   (b) thin filaments
   (c) sarcomeres
   (d) myosin crossbridges

2. What is the "trigger mechanism" for the sliding filament process?
   (a) the release of calcium ions
   (b) the release of adenosine triphosphate (ATP)
   (c) the release of troponin
   (d) the release of tropomyosin

3. The process from the initial nerve impulse through to the final muscle contraction is known as
   (a) the knee-jerk response
   (b) the actin-myosin interaction
   (c) excitation-contraction coupling
   (d) none of the above

4. Three types of muscle contraction are
   (a) afferent, intermediate, and efferent
   (b) chemical, electrical, and mechanical
   (c) autonomic, automatic, and somatic
   (d) concentric, eccentric, and isometric

5. Sensory receptors within a muscle fibre that primarily detect changes in muscle length are
   (a) intrafusal muscle fibres
   (b) muscle spindles
   (c) sensory neurons
   (d) motor neurons

6. Golgi tendon organs (GTOs) are sensory receptors at the end of muscle fibres that detect changes in
   (a) muscle tension
   (b) muscle length
   (c) muscle movement
   (d) muscle strength

Short-Answer Questions

MISSION: Briefly answer the following questions in the space provided:

1. What is meant by the "reflex arc"?

2. What are two important roles of the stretch reflex?

3. As a kind of tension detection device for the muscle system, what protective role do GTOs play?

Essay Questions

MISSION: On a separate piece of paper, develop a 100-word response to the following questions.

1. Describe the sliding filament theory of muscle contraction.

2. Explain in general terms how the proprioceptor system plays an indispensable role in bodily movement.

3. Compare and contrast monosynaptic reflexes and polysynaptic reflexes.

My Notes on Chapter 6

Use the space below to make notes on the questions on the facing page, to record any thoughts and ideas you have on this chapter, and to store study tips to help you prepare for tests and exams.

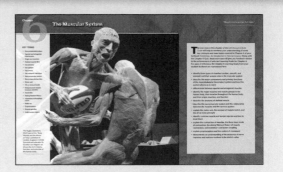

Chapter 6 Review (Student Textbook page 207)

Knowledge

1. Describe the major components and primary functions of the musculoskeletal system and explain how this system allows us to move.

2. Explain why muscles are typically arranged as opposing pairs. Give some examples of opposing muscles and muscle groups and the movements they allow.

3. Define the following terms: (a) neuromuscular system; (b) neuromuscular junction; (c) motor unit; (d) motor neuron; and e) the all-or-none principle.

4. Describe the sliding filament theory of muscle contraction in terms that anyone could understand.

5. Define the term "reflex" and state the differences between (a) a cerebral reflex and a spinal reflex; and (b) autonomic reflexes and somatic reflexes.

6. List the five parts of a reflex arc.

7. Identify the muscle or muscle group responsible for the following functions: (a) facial expression; (b) the body's upright position; (c) breathing; (d) flexion and rotation of the vertebral column; (e) movements of the wrist; (f) knee extension and hip flexion.

8. Rotator cuff tears are an occupational hazard for baseball pitchers. These muscles are commonly referred to as the S.I.T.S. or S.S.I.T. muscles. What do these acronyms stand for?

Thinking and Inquiry

9. Muscles "pull," they never "push." Elaborate on this distinction in the context of the three types of muscle contraction (concentric, eccentric, and isometric).

10. Differentiate between the terms "origin" and "insertion" in relation to a skeletal muscle and give an example of how each of these points of attachment functions during movement of a major muscle or muscle group.

11. A friend began a rigorous new exercise program several days ago and is worried about pain and swelling around a muscle. What can you tell your friend to provide reassurance that the pain and swelling are probably temporary?

12. Identify what you interpret to be the most complex muscle or muscle group in the human body, and elaborate on your thinking.

13. Select a muscle or muscle group that interests you (perhaps one with an unusual name, such as "psoas minor"). Gather additional facts about this muscle or muscle group—including how it got its name, its origin and insertion, and its function or functions. Write up a brief summary of your findings and present it in class.

Communication

14. Sketch two cross-sectional drawings showing the anatomy of skeletal muscle, first looking outward from the surface of the individual muscle fibre and then looking inward at the layers of tissue that make up the muscle fibre itself. Now develop a mnemonic aid or a phrase that will help you recall these layers of muscle tissue.

15. Design a flow chart to represent the process by which a muscle contracts (i.e., the sliding filament theory), beginning with the "trigger mechanism."

16. Draw a graphic organizer that maps out the major components of the human nervous system and how they relate to one another. Highlight the component that is primarily responsible for muscle action.

Application

17. Tendonitis is typically the result of overuse of muscles during repeated tennis strokes or golf swings. How would you explain "tennis tendonitis" or "golfer's elbow" to a person who has suffered this injury? Which muscles and tendons are affected in each case, and what is the generally prescribed treatment?

18. The process of muscle contraction as a whole is sometimes described as "excitation-contraction coupling," a process that happens in an instant. Using an example of a muscle movement (e.g., raising your hand in class), write out in point form the sequence of steps involved in this process, from the initial nerve impulse to the muscle contraction.

19. Invent a new game that will help you and your classmates recall the names of the major muscles and muscle groups of the body, as well as the origin, insertion, and function of these muscles.

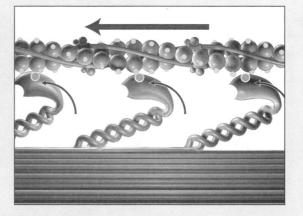

The mechanism of the sliding filament theory of muscle contraction. The process of muscle contraction as a whole is often referred to as "excitation-contraction coupling."

Energy Systems and Physical Activity

KEY TERMS

- Essential nutrients
- Carbohydrates
- Glycogen
- Adenosine triphosphate (ATP)
- Anaerobic system
- Aerobic system
- ATP-PC system
- Glycolysis
- Lactic acid
- Cellular respiration
- Fats
- Protein
- Slow-twitch muscle fibres
- Fast-twitch muscle fibres
- Myoglobin

Meghan Agosta-Marciano has represented Canada at the 2006 Winter Olympics in Turin, the 2010 Winter Olympics in Vancouver, and the 2014 Winter Olympics in Sochi, winning gold medals at all three.

Lurii Osadchi/Shutterstock

The exercises in this chapter of the *Lab Manual & Study Guide* will help to reinforce your understanding of some key concepts and main topics covered in Chapter 7 of your textbook *Kinesiology: An Introduction to Exercise Science.* Along with the Chapter 7 Quiz, these exercises will give you feedback related to the achievement of selected Learning Goals for Chapter 7. For ease of reference, the Chapter 7 Learning Goals from your student textbook are reproduced here:

- describe three key energy nutrients (carbohydrates, fats, and proteins) and the reconstitution of ATP (the common energy molecule) within our bodies to produce energy

- differentiate between two energy systems in our bodies: anaerobic (without oxygen) and aerobic (with oxygen)

- explain the basic processes and functions of the body's three metabolic pathways within the two energy systems: ATP-PC (anaerobic alactic); glycolysis (anaerobic lactic), and cellular respiration

- identify the role of pyruvate (pyruvic acid) and lactic acid in glycolysis and describe the effects of lactic acid buildup

- differentiate between slow-twitch and fast-twitch muscle fibre types, including the relative amount of myoglobin each type contains, and describe their roles in human muscular activity

- describe the functions and distribution of Type I, Type IIA, and Type IIB muscle fibre types

- analyze the relationship between muscle fibre type and athletic performance, including the different physiological demands imposed by particular sports

- explain how an athlete should match training methods to energy needs to maximize performance

- contrast how the body uses fats and proteins as energy sources with how the body uses carbohydrates/glucose sources to produce energy from ATP

WORKSHEET

7.1 Two Energy Systems, Three Metabolic Pathways

There are two energy systems (anaerobic and aerobic) but three "metabolic pathways." This worksheet will help you distinguish these pathways and assist you in remembering how human energy systems work.

Name: _____

Date: _____

MISSION: The three metabolic energy pathways intersect and overlap continuously in all types of physical activity. Below, however, are photographs of athletes in three different sports that tend to rely more heavily on one of the three metabolic pathways over the others. In the space below each photograph, list other sports and physical activities that would rely heavily on one of the three pathways compared to the other two.

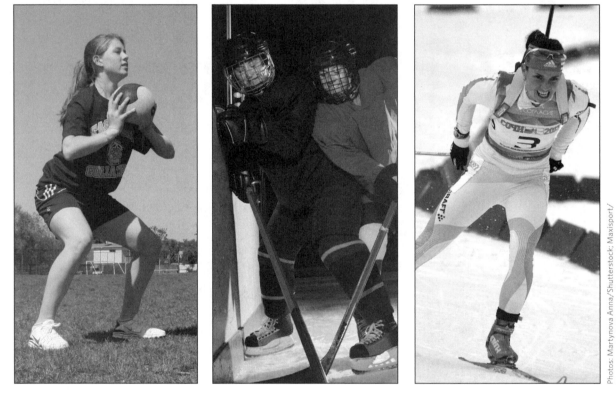

Photos: Martynova Anna/Shutterstock; Maxisport/Shutterstock; CLS Design/Shutterstock

1: The ATP/PC System (Anaerobic Alactic)

_____
_____
_____
_____
_____
_____
_____

2: Glycolysis (Anaerobic Lactic)

_____
_____
_____
_____
_____
_____
_____

3: Cellular Respiration (Aerobic)

_____
_____
_____
_____
_____
_____
_____

MISSION: Examine the illustrations of the three metabolic energy pathways below. Explain what is happening in your own words.

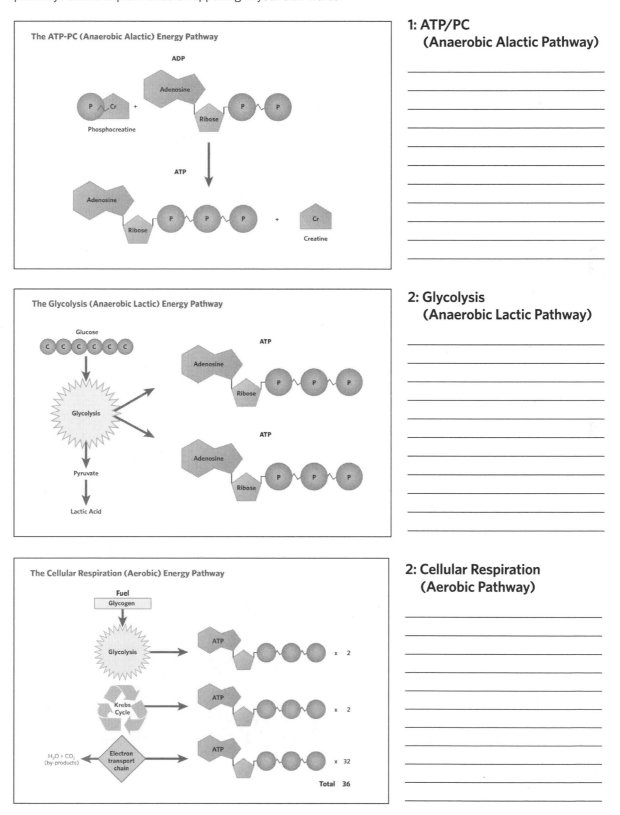

1: ATP/PC
(Anaerobic Alactic Pathway)

_____
_____
_____
_____
_____
_____
_____
_____
_____
_____
_____
_____

2: Glycolysis
(Anaerobic Lactic Pathway)

_____
_____
_____
_____
_____
_____
_____
_____
_____
_____
_____
_____

2: Cellular Respiration
(Aerobic Pathway)

_____
_____
_____
_____
_____
_____
_____
_____
_____
_____
_____
_____

WORKSHEET

7.2 The Three Energy Pathways Compared

ATP-PC (the anaerobic alactic pathway), glycolysis (the anaerobic lactic pathway), and cellular respiration (the aerobic pathway) are the three basic energy pathways that supply the energy needed for working muscles.

Name: _____

Date: _____

MISSION: Fill in the following table based on the criteria provided in the left-hand column.

A Comparison of the Three Energy Pathways within the Human Body			
	ATP-PC (Anaerobic alactic pathway)	**Glycolysis** (Anaerobic lactic pathway)	**Cellular Respiration** (Aerobic pathway)
Location of activity			
Energy source			
Uses oxygen or not			
ATP produced			
Duration			
Number of chemical reactions			
By-products			
Basic chemical reaction formula			
Type of activities			
Types of exercise that rely on this system			
Advantages			
Limitation of energy system			

7.3 Energy Pathways and Athletic Performance

Every sport or activity involves the use of the three energy pathways to varying degrees, depending on the sport's unique requirements. Some sports rely more heavily on one pathway while others use a combination of all three.

Name: _____

Date: _____

MISSION: Complete the following chart by indicating the extent (expressed as a percentage or as "highly," "moderately," or "seldom used") to which the activities listed below rely on each of the three energy pathways. In the remaining spaces in the left-hand column, choose as many additional sports as you can and provide the same information in the corresponding columns.

Energy Systems For Various Sports			
Sport or Activity	ATP-PC (Anaerobic Alactic Pathway)	Glycolysis (Anaerobic Lactic Pathway)	Cellular Respiration (Aerobic Pathway)
Olympic weightlifting			
Endurance running			
100-metre sprint			
A 30-second shift in hockey			

WORKSHEET

Chapter 7 Quiz

The two sets of questions below will test your knowledge and broaden your understanding of the material covered in Chapter 7. Complete each set of questions according to your teacher's instructions.

Name: _____

Date: _____

Question Set 1: Energy Sources and Energy Systems in the Human Body

Multiple-Choice Questions

MISSION: Circle the letter beside the answer that you believe to be correct.

1. To be usable as sources of energy, the nutrients (proteins, fats, and especially carbohydrates) in our food must be resynthesized in our bodies into
   (a) adenosine triphosphate (ATP)
   (b) glycogen
   (c) phosphocreatine
   (d) phosphate

2. Which of the following sport activities primarily use the ATP-PC system?
   (a) circuit training
   (b) shot put
   (c) 400-metre sprint
   (d) all of the above

3. Which of the following is the main product of glycolysis?
   (a) acetyl CoA
   (b) pyruvate
   (c) ADP
   (d) creatine phosphate

4. Cellular respiration involves which of the following energy sub-pathways?
   (a) glycolysis
   (b) Krebs cycle
   (c) electron transport chain
   (d) all of the above

5. Upon which energy system does a marathon runner rely heavily?
   (a) ATP-PC
   (b) glycolysis
   (c) cellular respiration
   (d) none of the above

6. During physical exercise, our bodies' primary sources of energy are
   (a) proteins and fats
   (b) proteins and carbohydrates
   (c) carbohydrates and fats
   (d) none of the above

Short-Answer Questions

MISSION: Briefly answer the following questions in the space provided:

1. What are the three metabolic pathways by which energy from ATP is produced for use in our bodies?

2. Under certain conditions, glycolysis could be considered the first stage of cellular respiration. What are these conditions?

3. What is "lactic acid buildup" and why is it sometimes a problem for athletes?

Essay Questions

MISSION: On a separate piece of paper, develop a 100-word response to the following questions.

1. Identify the body's two main energy systems, describe the three metabolic pathways within those systems, and state the factors that place limits on each of these pathways.

2. During which types of sports and performance events does the anaerobic lactic system contribute little energy? Why is this so?

3. Each energy pathway results in different quantities of ATP. How much ATP is associated with each pathway? Explain.

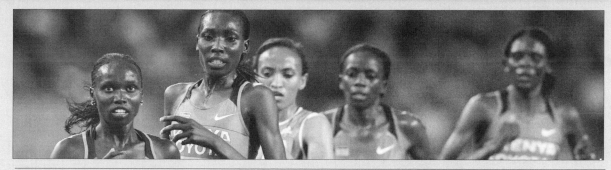

AP Photo/Lee Jin-man

Question Set 2: Muscle Fibre Types and Human Performance

Multiple-Choice Questions

MISSION: Circle the letter beside the answer that you believe to be correct.

1. Slow-twitch muscle fibres contain high amounts of this oxygen storage unit.
   (a) hemoglobin
   (b) myosin ATPase
   (c) alanine
   (d) myoglobin

2. Fast-twitch muscle fibres
   (a) are red/dark in colour; tense and relax slowly
   (b) are pale in colour; tense and relax quickly
   (c) can activate at a rate two to three times faster than slow-twitch muscle fibres
   (d) (b) and (c) are correct

3. Which of the following muscles are likely to contain a large amount of fast-twitch fibres?
   (a) quadriceps
   (b) erector spinae
   (c) hamstrings
   (d) eyelids

4. Which type of muscle fibre do exercise physiologists believe can be modified as a consequence of aerobic endurance training?
   (a) Type I or Slow Oxidative (SO)
   (b) Type IIA or Fast-Oxidative Glycolytic (FOG)
   (c) Type IIB or Fast-Glycolytic (FG)
   (d) none of the above

5. Which of the following non-physiological factors could be associated with the remarkable achievement of East African distance runners?
   (a) unique local customs and culture
   (b) the example set by other East African athletes
   (c) potential financial gain for their families
   (d) all of the above

6. Which female African distance runner won gold in the 10,000-m race at the 2012 London Olympics?
   (a) Ethiopia's Triunesh Dibaba
   (b) Kenya's Vivian Cheruiyot
   (c) Ethiopia's Meseret Defar
   (d) Kenya's Linet Masai

Short-Answer Questions

MISSION: Briefly answer the following questions in the space provided:

1. Describe the characteristics of fast-twitch and slow-twitch muscle fibres.

2. Explain the role of the protein myoglobin with respect to muscle fibre types.

3. Exercise physiologists distinguish an "intermediate" muscle fibre type. What is unique about this particular muscle fibre type?

Essay Questions

MISSION: On a separate piece of paper, develop a 100-word response to the following questions.

1. Draw up a table that lists and compares the characteristics of slow-twitch and fast-twitch muscle fibre.

2. East African distance runners win a disproportionate number of endurance races. Describe some factors that might account for their successes.

3. Explain why training at high altitude may help endurance athletes when they compete at sea level.

WORKSHEET

My Notes on Chapter 7

Use the space below to make notes on the questions on the facing page, to record any thoughts and ideas you have on this chapter, and to store study tips to help you prepare for tests and exams.

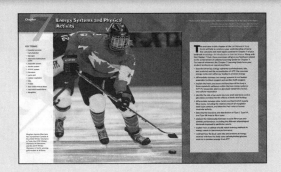

_____   _____

_____   _____

_____   _____

_____   _____

_____   _____

_____   _____

_____   _____

_____   _____

_____   _____

_____   _____

_____   _____

_____   _____

_____   _____

_____   _____

_____   _____

_____   _____

_____   _____

_____   _____

_____   _____

_____   _____

_____   _____

_____   _____

_____   _____

_____   _____

_____   _____

_____   _____

Chapter 7 Review (Student Textbook page 229)

Knowledge

1. The energy our bodies use comes directly from the nutrients in the food we eat, especially carbohydrates. Into which universal form of energy are these nutrients reconstituted for use in muscle contraction and other physiological processes? Describe the final form of this common form of energy at the molecular level.

2. List and briefly describe the two energy systems and the three metabolic pathways by means of which ATP energy reserves are restored in the body.

3. The two anaerobic energy pathways are sometimes referred to as "lactic" and "alactic." Write a clear definition for each of these terms.

4. All sports generally involve all three metabolic pathways, but often one pathway can be considered the predominant one for that sport. For each of the three metabolic pathways, list three examples of sports that rely primarily on that pathway.

5. Exercise physiologists distinguish between two general types of muscle fibre. Identify each type and state the main differences between them.

6. Match each of the two general types of muscle fibre to three different sports or physical activities.

7. Identify which muscle fibre type is (a) more fatigue-resistant, and which muscle fibre type (b) allows for more generation of force over a short period of time.

8. In terms of training, what general strategy can an athlete adopt to maximize performance? Give two or three examples to support your answer.

Thinking and Inquiry

9. Break down the various bioenergetic processes that glucose undergoes in our bodies, from the assimilation of carbohydrates in the food we eat to the use of glucose as an energy source for physical activity.

10. Under certain conditions, glycolysis (the second metabolic pathway) becomes the first stage of the cellular respiration pathway. What are the conditions that must be present for this to happen? What will be the likely outcome if these conditions are not present?

11. In relation to energy production, which kinds of training activities do you think might be most beneficial for a shot putter, a tennis player, and a marathon runner? Which kinds of training activities would likely be least beneficial in each case? Explain your answer.

12. Slow-twitch muscle fibre is commonly described as being reddish in colour, whereas fast-twitch muscle fibre is more whitish. What might account for this difference in colour? Provide an example or two in your response.

Communication

13. Chemical equations are a shorthand way to describe what is happening during a chemical reaction. Work in groups of three, with each person selecting one metabolic pathway. Each student takes turns presenting and explaining the chemical equation that represents the chosen metabolic pathway to the other two students in the group.

14. Cellular respiration, which is the third metabolic pathway, involves three complex sub-pathways, yielding large amounts of ATP. Prepare a slideshow presentation that identifies each sub-pathway (starting with glycolysis), the number of ATP molecules produced in each sub-pathway, and the by-products of each sub-pathway.

15. Create a point-form fact sheet on the topic of muscle fibre types and energy systems that could be posted to the website of a personal training facility.

Application

16. Create a table that lists the three metabolic pathways in rows and that features a column for each of the following: ATP Yield, Requires Glucose, Requires Oxygen, Yields Lactic Acid, Limiting Factors. Fill in the table with the required information in each cell.

17. Categorize which muscle fibre types and which energy systems are activated at each stage of a triathlon.

18. At one time, obstacles to obtaining dead bodies (cadavers) and obtaining legal permission to dissect them prevented scientists from understanding basic anatomy and physiology. Prepare a short report on ethical issues that might arise in conducting research into muscle-fibre types in humans or animals.

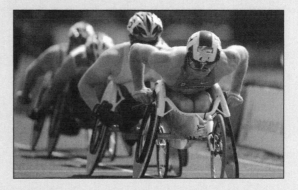

A great many factors, apart from biological and physiological make-up, contribute to helping an individual excel at a chosen sport. Ottawa's John Cassidy wins the 80-metre wheelchair race in Manchester, England, 2012. (AP Photo/Jon Super)

The Cardiovascular and Respiratory Systems

KEY TERMS

- Myocardium
- Pulmonary circulation
- Systemic circulation
- Sinoatrial node (SA node)
- Atrioventricular node (AV node)
- Arteries
- Arterioles
- Capillaries
- Veins
- Cardiac output (Q)
- Heart rate
- Cardiac cycle
- Systolic and diastolic blood pressure
- External respiration
- Internal respiration
- Conductive zone
- Respiratory zone
- Diffusion
- O_2 transport
- CO_2 transport
- Pulmonary ventilation (V_E)
- a-vO_2 diff
- Asthma
- Chronic obstructive pulmonary disease (COPD)
- Maximal rate of oxygen consumption (VO$_2$max)
- Oxygen deficit (O_2 deficit)
- Ventilatory threshold
- Lactate threshold

The peloton makes its way up Mount Royal at the Grand Prix Cycliste de Montréal in 2011. The cyclists form a group (a peloton) by riding close to other riders in order to save energy ("drafting" or "slipstreaming").

Meunierd/Shutterstock

> **"Trust no thought arrived at while sitting down."**
> — Long-distance running expert Dr. George Sheehan

The exercises in this chapter of the *Lab Manual & Study Guide* will help to reinforce your understanding of some key concepts and main topics covered in Chapter 8 of your textbook *Kinesiology: An Introduction to Exercise Science.* Along with the Chapter 8 Quiz, these exercises will give you feedback related to the achievement of selected Learning Goals for Chapter 8. For ease of reference, the Chapter 8 Learning Goals from your student textbook are reproduced here:

- describe the basic structure and function of the cardiovascular system (the heart, blood vessels, and blood)
- describe the circulation (path) of blood through the heart
- describe the heart's cardiac muscle contractions and the electrical excitation of the heart
- explain the role of the vascular system (arteries, arterioles, capillaries, veins, blood) within the cardiovascular system
- describe several cardiovascular diseases and their causes, risks, and cures
- describe the cardiovascular system's response to exercise, e.g., cardiac output, heart rate, and blood pressure
- analyze the effects of training on the cardiovascular system
- describe the basic function and structure of the respiratory system and its importance to the body's overall function
- differentiate between the two basic zones (conductive and respiratory) of the respiratory system
- describe the mechanisms of breathing (ventilation)
- describe the body's system of gas exchange
- describe various respiratory dynamics that occur during exercise and identify two common respiratory diseases
- describe the integration of cardiovascular and respiratory functions, including maximal rate of oxygen consumption
- explain the causes of oxygen deficit and blood lactate accumulation during the rest-to-exercise transition

WORKSHEET

8.1 The Anterior Structure of the Heart

The anterior view of the heart reveals the major structures of the heart: the coronary vessels (the coronary arteries and the coronary veins), and the four separate chambers that make up the heart.

Name: _____

Date: _____

MISSION: Label the illustration below using the list of labels provided.

Labels

- ❏ Anterior interventricular branch of left coronary artery
- ❏ Aorta
- ❏ Branches of left pulmonary artery
- ❏ Branches of right pulmonary artery
- ❏ Great cardiac vein

- ❏ Inferior vena cava
- ❏ Left atrium
- ❏ Left pulmonary artery
- ❏ Left pulmonary veins
- ❏ Left ventricle
- ❏ Pulmonary trunk
- ❏ Right atrium

- ❏ Right coronary artery
- ❏ Right pulmonary veins
- ❏ Right ventricle
- ❏ Small cardiac vein
- ❏ Superior vena cava
- ❏ Thoracic aorta (descending)

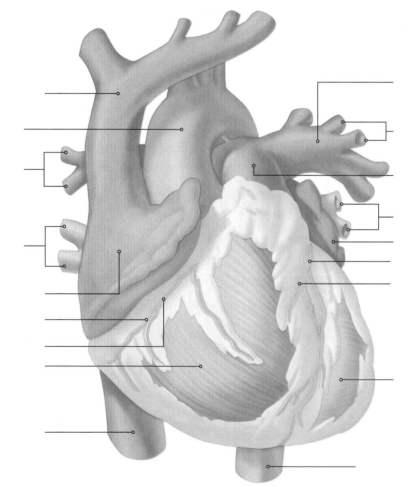

Anterior view of the coronary vessels, including other major heart structures.

WORKSHEET

8.2 The Flow of Blood within the Heart

The heart is a complex organ formed from specialized muscle tissue called myocardium. The heart acts as the "pump" of the cardiovascular system, pushing blood through the blood vessels throughout the body.

Name: _____

Date: _____

MISSION: To gain familiarity with the heart's key internal components, label the illustration below. Some labels may need to be used more than once. Next, colour parts of the heart and the arrows to indicate the circulation of oxygenated blood (red) and deoxygenated blood (blue) throughout the heart.

Labels

- ❏ Aortic semilunar valve
- ❏ Bicuspid (mitral) valve
- ❏ Chordae tendinae
- ❏ Interventricular septum

- ❏ Left atrium
- ❏ Left ventricle
- ❏ Papillary muscles
- ❏ Pulmonary semilunar valve

- ❏ Right atrium
- ❏ Right pulmonary veins
- ❏ Right ventricle
- ❏ Tricuspid valve

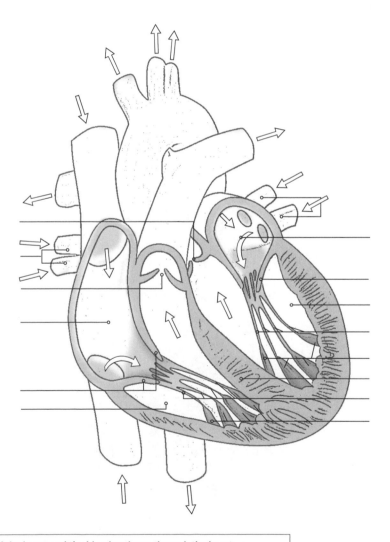

Internal anatomy of the heart and the blood pathway through the heart.

WORKSHEET

8.3 The Electrical Conduction System of the Heart

The electrical conduction system of the heart is an intricate and continuous system that allows the heart to function properly. Cardiac muscle cells are interconnected and allow the passage of electrical signals from cell to cell.

Name: _____

Date: _____

MISSION: To gain a better understanding of the processes involved in the heart's electrical conduction system and to identify the components involved in this system, label the illustration below and colour the nerves (using a yellow marker or pencil crayon).

Labels

- ❏ Atrioventricular (AV) node
- ❏ Bundle of His (AV bundle)
- ❏ Internodal pathways
- ❏ Purkinje fibres
- ❏ Right and left bundle branches
- ❏ Sinoatrial (SA) node

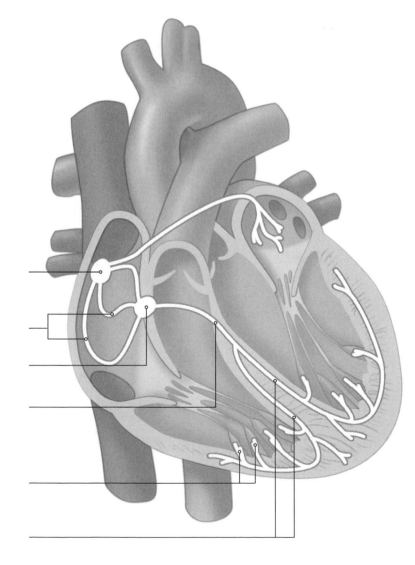

The electrical conduction system of the heart.

WORKSHEET

8.4 The Structure of the Cardiovascular System

The cardiovascular system is comprised of large and small blood vessels. Oxygenated blood goes out to the body from the heart and deoxygenated blood flows back to the heart, and then to the lungs.

Name: _____

Date: _____

MISSION: To gain a better understanding of the components and function of the essential structure of the cardiovascular system, label the illustration below. Note the arrows indicating the direction of the flow of blood as you are labelling the illustration.

Labels

- ❏ Arteriole
- ❏ Capillaries
- ❏ Capillary bed
- ❏ Large arteries
- ❏ Large veins
- ❏ Medium arteries
- ❏ Medium veins
- ❏ Venules

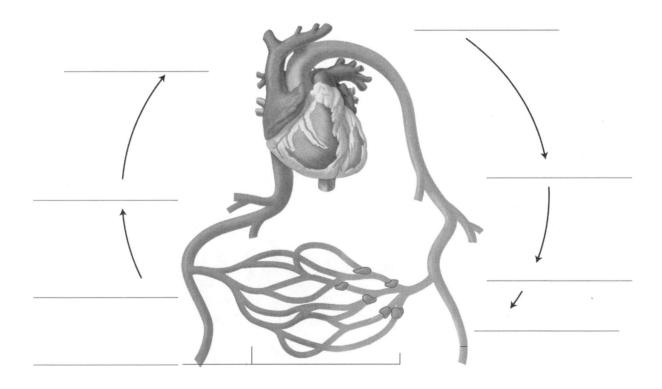

The cardiovascular system.

WORKSHEET

8.5 The Structure of the Respiratory System

The respiratory system is composed of many interconnected parts that allow the passage of air. The structure of the respiratory system can be divided into two main zones: the conductive zone and the respiratory zone.

Name: _____

Date: _____

MISSION: Label the illustration below using the list of labels provided, and indicate the two main structures.

Labels

- ❏ Alveolar sacs
- ❏ Alveoli
- ❏ Conductive zone
- ❏ Epiglottis
- ❏ Larynx
- ❏ Left and right primary bronchi
- ❏ Left lung (2 lobes)

- ❏ Mouth
- ❏ Nasal cavity
- ❏ Pulmonary arteriole (carrying deoxygenated blood)
- ❏ Pulmonary venule (carrying oxygenated blood)
- ❏ Respiratory zone

- ❏ Right lung (3 lobes)
- ❏ Smooth muscle
- ❏ Terminal bronchiole
- ❏ Trachea

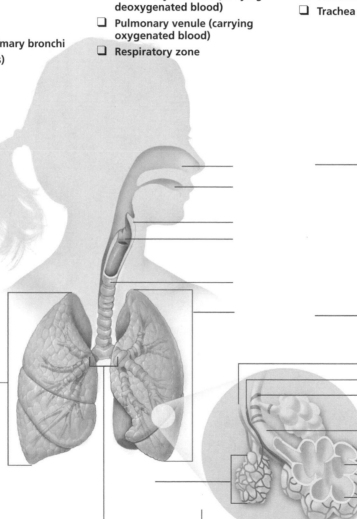

The main structures of the respiratory system.

WORKSHEET

8.6 External and Internal Respiration

External respiration involves the exchange of O_2 and CO_2 in the lungs. Internal respiration refers to the exchange of gases at the tissue level where CO_2 is delivered and CO_2 is removed from the blood.

Name: _____

Date: _____

MISSION: To gain a better understanding of the structure and function of the external and internal respiration pathways, label the illustration below. Some labels may need to be used more than once. Next, colour the oxygenated blood (red) and the deoxygenated blood (blue) to demonstrate blood flow.

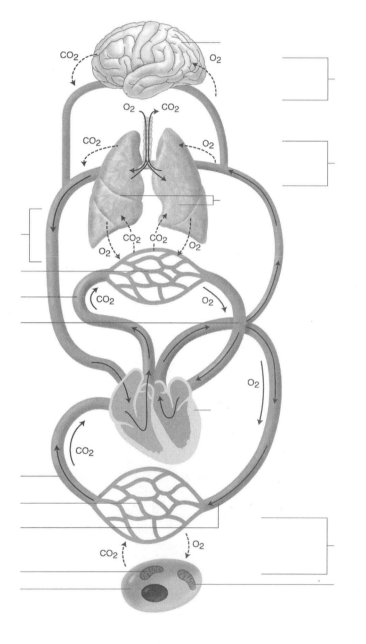

Labels

- ❑ Brain
- ❑ Cellular respiration
- ❑ External respiration
- ❑ Heart
- ❑ Internal respiration
- ❑ Lungs
- ❑ Mitochondria
- ❑ Pulmonary arteries
- ❑ Pulmonary capillaries
- ❑ Pulmonary veins
- ❑ Systemic arteries
- ❑ Systemic capillaries
- ❑ Systemic veins
- ❑ Tissue cell

External and internal respiration in the human body.

WORKSHEET

Chapter 8 Quiz

The two sets of questions below will test your knowledge and broaden your understanding of the material covered in Chapter 8. Complete each set of questions according to your teacher's instructions.

Name: _____

Date: _____

Question Set 1: The Cardiovascular System—Structure and Function

Multiple-Choice Questions

MISSION: Circle the letter beside the answer that you believe to be correct.

1. Which of the following blood vessels drains the head, the neck, and the arms?
   (a) the pulmonary artery
   (b) the inferior vena cava
   (c) the superior vena cava
   (d) the aorta

2. The bicuspid (mitral) valve is located between
   (a) the right ventricle and the pulmonary artery
   (b) the left ventricle and the aorta
   (c) the left atrium and the left ventricle
   (d) the right atrium and the right ventricle

3. Which of the following blood vessels carries deoxygenated blood from the heart to the lungs?
   (a) the pulmonary vein
   (b) the coronary arteries
   (c) the aorta
   (d) the pulmonary artery

4. This structure in the heart is sometimes referred to as the heart's "pacemaker."
   (a) the pulmonary semilunar valve
   (b) the myocardium
   (c) the atrioventricular (AV) node
   (d) the sinoatrial (SA) node

5. Cardiac output is equal to which of the following?
   (a) heart rate x breathing rate
   (b) heart rate x stroke volume
   (c) heart rate x aortic blood pressure
   (d) resting heart rate

6. Which of the following remains unaffected with respect to blood distribution during exercise?
   (a) the brain
   (b) the digestive system
   (c) the skeletal muscle
   (d) the muscular system

Short-Answer Questions

MISSION: Briefly answer the following questions in the space provided:

1. What are the three main tools, or systems, that the body uses to assist in the return of blood in the veins back to the heart?

2. What are the main components of human blood?

3. What is meant by systolic and diastolic blood pressure?

Essay Questions

MISSION: On a separate piece of paper, develop a 100-word response to the following questions.

1. Trace the path of blood through the heart, briefly explaining the role of each component of the cardiovascular system.

2. Discuss several risk factors that may lead to coronary heart disease, and suggest ways to offset such disease.

3. What are some distinguishing characteristics of an elite athlete's heart?

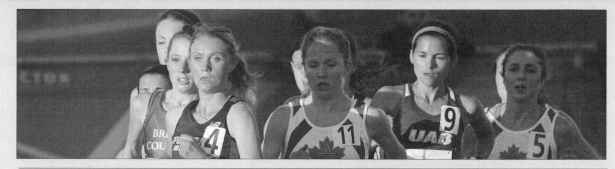

Jamie Roach/Shutterstock

Question Set 2: The Cardiorespiratory System—Structure and Function

Multiple-Choice Questions

MISSION: Circle the letter beside the answer that you believe to be correct.

1. The respiratory zone is composed of the
   (a) pharynx, trachea, and respiratory bronchioles
   (b) mouth, nose, bronchi, and alveolar sacs
   (c) trachea, bronchi, bronchioles, and alveolar ducts
   (d) respiratory bronchioles, alveolar ducts, and alveolar sacs

2. As the diaphragm contracts, the thoracic cavity
   (a) tightens and shrinks
   (b) pulls downwards and enlarges
   (c) remains fairly stationary and in place
   (d) recoils to its original position

3. The smallest vessels in the cardiovascular system that are responsible for the exchange of gases are
   (a) arteries
   (b) veins
   (c) arterioles
   (d) capillaries

4. The maximal amount of O_2 that can be taken in and used for the metabolic production of ATP during exercise is known as
   (a) O_2 uptake
   (b) VCO_2
   (c) VO_2max
   (d) RER

5. The difference between the oxygen required to perform a task and the oxygen actually consumed prior to reaching a new steady state is known as the
   (a) CO_2 deficit
   (b) a-vO_2 diff
   (c) O_2 deficit
   (d) OBLA

6. The point where blood lactate concentrations begin to increase is referred to as
   (a) the ventilatory threshold
   (b) excess post-exercise oxygen consumption
   (c) blood lactate accumulation
   (d) the lactate threshold

Short-Answer Questions

MISSION: Briefly answer the following questions in the space provided:

1. With reference to the cardiorespiratory system, what is meant by the "conductive zone"?

2. What is meant by "external respiration" and "internal respiration"?

3. What does "a-vO_2 diff" refer to?

Essay Questions

MISSION: On a separate piece of paper, develop a 100-word response to the following questions.

1. Describe the mechanisms of breathing.

2. Describe the factors that affect gas exchange (the rates of diffusion of O_2 and CO_2 at the lungs and the tissues).

3. Explain what is meant by VO_2max and what factors affect it.

4. Identify and describe the kinds of diseases that can affect the respiratory system.

WORKSHEET

My Notes on Chapter 8

Use the space below to make notes on the questions on the facing page, to record any thoughts and ideas you have on this chapter, and to store study tips to help you prepare for tests and exams.

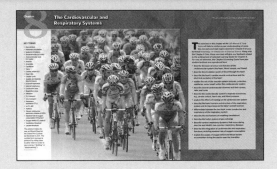

Chapter 8 Review (Student Textbook page 267)

Knowledge

1. Exercise physiologists distinguish between pulmonary circulation and systemic circulation. Explain how the two systems differ from one another.
2. The electrical conduction system of the heart relies on two specialized regions of tissue, or nodes. Name these two nodes and describe the main function of each one.
3. A normal blood pressure reading is in the range of 120/80 (stated as "120 over 80"). Explain what these two numbers represent.
4. During exercise, the cardiovascular system alters the blood flow distribution throughout the body. Explain why this is the case, giving examples.
5. Exercise physiologists divide the respiratory system into the conductive zone and the respiratory zone. Describe the different structures that make up each zone and then explain the functions of each zone.
6. Describe the basic mechanisms involved in breathing with respect to sequence of muscle contractions and air pressure differentials.
7. VO_2max is the most commonly used measure of aerobic fitness. In your own words, explain this concept.
8. Explain how three different body systems can potentially limit VO2max.

Thinking and Inquiry

9. Compare and contrast skeletal muscle with cardiac muscle in terms of structure and function. Highlight the unique characteristics of cardiac muscle that keep our hearts beating.
10. Using a graphic organizer of your choice, summarize the various factors involved in the body's cardiovascular dynamics (i.e., how the cardiovascular system adapts to accommodate the ever-changing demands placed on it).
11. Identify one major organ that is unaffected by the shift in blood flow distribution that occurs during exercise. Why do you think the amount of blood delivered to this organ is maintained both at rest and during exercise?
12. Summarize how various characteristics of the respiratory system maximize the rate of diffusion of O_2 from the air inhaled in the lungs into the blood, as well as the movement of CO_2 out of the blood.
13. Compare and contrast oxygen (O_2) transport in the blood with carbon dioxide (CO_2) transport in the blood.
14. "Individuals can increase their aerobic capacity through proper aerobic training." Elaborate on this statement by referring explicitly to varying oxygen deficits.

Communication

15. Create a drawing that shows the main structures of the heart. Overlay the drawing with a sketch (drawn on acetate or see-through paper) that traces the circulation of blood through the heart. Use color codes to indicate oxygenated and deoxygenated blood.
16. Exercise physiologists use the term a-vO2diff to refer to the amounts of O2 delivered to working muscles during exercise. Create your own graphic to illustrate the concept of a-vO2diff and how it is measured.
17. Create a table showing the possible effects of exercise on ventilatory threshold, a-vO2diff, and blood lactate concentration. Use plus or minus signs to indicate the direction of changes in each factor resulting from exercise.

Application

18. Develop a pamphlet (either print or online) to distribute throughout your school or community that explains primary causes of coronary disease and that lists ways to reduce the known risk factors associated with diseases of the heart and blood vessels.
19. As a class project, make a poster showing all the possible effects of exercise on the cardiovascular system (e.g., heart size, stroke volume, heart rate, number of capillaries, thickness of coronary arteries, blood volume, blood flow redistribution, blood flow to the brain). Use a series of plus and minus signs to indicate changes in each variable resulting from exercise.
20. Propose some measures that could be undertaken to increase public awareness of how to maintain a healthy respiratory system.

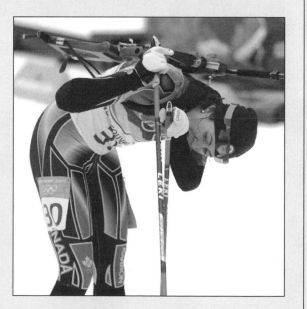

Megan Imrie, of Falcon Lake, Manitoba, "catches her breath" at the finish line of the gruelling 7.5 km biathlon sprint at the 2010 Vancouver Olympic Winter Games. (CP Photo/Boris Minkevich)

Career Choices

Investigate a career in one of the fields mentioned in this unit. Ideally, you should interview someone working within the field for this assignment. You can ask him or her the following questions and a lot more as well.

Name: _____

Date: _____

MISSION: Answer the series of questions below in relation to the career you have selected. If you interviewed a person for this career information, use quotation marks to distinguish what they said from your own comments on the career. Give the person's name and job title.

1 Career and description

_____

_____

_____

_____

_____

2 List at least two post-secondary institutions in Ontario and/or Canada that offer programs for this career.

_____

_____

_____

_____

3 Choose one of the above institutions and determine the required courses in the first year of study for this program.

_____

_____

_____

_____

_____

4 How many years of post-secondary education are required before beginning this career? Is an internship or apprenticeship required?

_____

_____

_____

_____

5 What is the demand for individuals qualified for this occupation? If possible, provide some employment data to support your answer.

_____

_____

_____

_____

6 What is the average starting salary for this career? What is the top salary? On what do salary increases depend in this career?

_____

_____

_____

_____

7 List occupational settings where a person with these qualifications could work.

_____

_____

_____

_____

Human Growth and Development

KEY TERMS

- Components of human growth and development
- Cephalocaudal sequence
- Proximodistal sequence
- Peak height velocity
- Critical periods
- Stages of human development
- Motor skill
- Canadian Society for Exercise Physiology (CSEP)
- Cognitive development
- Neuroscience
- Hippocampus
- Social and emotional development
- Friendship
- Long-Term Athlete Development (LTAD)
- LTAD growth tracking tables

An active and a health-conscious lifestyle fostered in childhood is likely to continue throughout a person's life. Here, seven- and eight-year-old children participate in a hockey tournament.

CP Photo/Richard Buchan

The exercises in this chapter of the *Lab Manual & Study Guide* will help to reinforce your understanding of some key concepts and main topics covered in Chapter 9 of your textbook *Kinesiology: An Introduction to Exercise Science.* Along with the Chapter 9 Quiz, these exercises will give you feedback related to the achievement of selected Learning Goals for Chapter 9. For ease of reference, the Chapter 9 Learning Goals from your student textbook are reproduced here:

• identify the four key components of growth and development (physical, cognitive, social, and emotional)

• describe the relationship between age and physical development, and the various ways of measuring age (chronological, skeletal, and developmental)

• describe observable patterns of growth and development and different rates of growth for different body parts, including the cephalocaudal and proximodistal sequences

• identify the four main stages of physical growth and development from infancy to adulthood and describe the factors that affect this development

• describe the influence of Jean Piaget's four-stage model of human cognitive development

• describe the correlation between physical activity and enhanced cognitive development

• identify factors in healthy social and emotional development, including the formation of friendships and participation in sport and recreational activities

• explain the importance of modifying physical activities and simplifying rules to match the developmental characteristics, ability levels, and skill levels of different age groups

• demonstrate an ability to design a movement-based activity appropriate to a particular age and stage of development

WORKSHEET

9.1 Factors Affecting Human Growth and Development

Human growth and development are complex processes involving several interrelated components. These components vary from one person to the next, and they all contribute to an individual's overall development.

Name: _____

Date: _____

The Four Components of Human Growth and Development: An Overview

MISSION: Review the graphic representation below, which shows the four components of human growth and development. On the next page, list the various factors that affect each of these components.

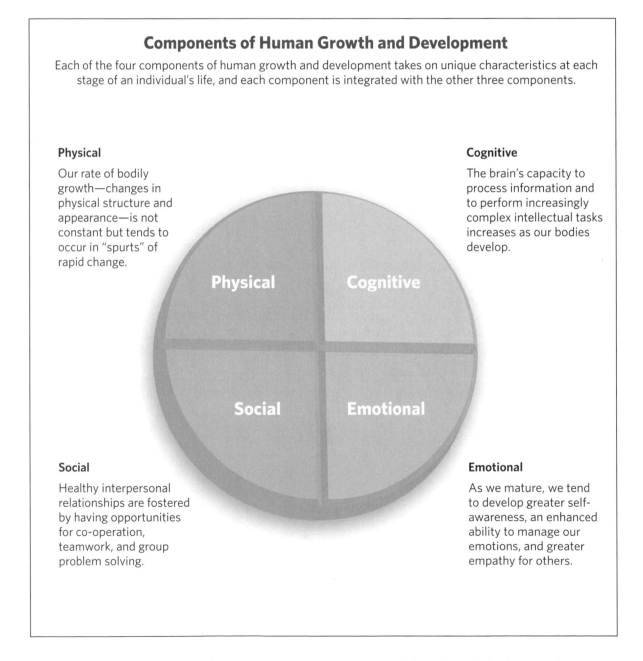

Components of Human Growth and Development

Each of the four components of human growth and development takes on unique characteristics at each stage of an individual's life, and each component is integrated with the other three components.

Physical

Our rate of bodily growth—changes in physical structure and appearance—is not constant but tends to occur in "spurts" of rapid change.

Cognitive

The brain's capacity to process information and to perform increasingly complex intellectual tasks increases as our bodies develop.

Social

Healthy interpersonal relationships are fostered by having opportunities for co-operation, teamwork, and group problem solving.

Emotional

As we mature, we tend to develop greater self-awareness, an enhanced ability to manage our emotions, and greater empathy for others.

Identifying Specific Factors Affecting Human Growth and Development

Work with a small group of classmates on this exercise. Referring to the graphic representation on the previous page, compile a list of the various factors that affect each component of human growth and development. For each component, list four key factors that exert an influence on that component.

Physical Component

Cognitive Component

Social Component

Emotional Component

☞ Look in the Book, pp. 272-289

WORKSHEET

9.2 Create Your Own Personal Development Timeline

Experts in the area of human growth and development sometimes speak of "developmental milestones"—significant events such as learning to walk and talk or making friendships for the first time.

Name: _____

Date: _____

MISSION: Fill in as much of the chart as possible to create your own personal development timeline. Record the most significant events, or milestones, in your physical, cognitive, social, and emotional development.

Ages	Physical Development	Cognitive Development
Ages 1-5		
Ages 6-10		
Ages 11-15		
Age 16+		

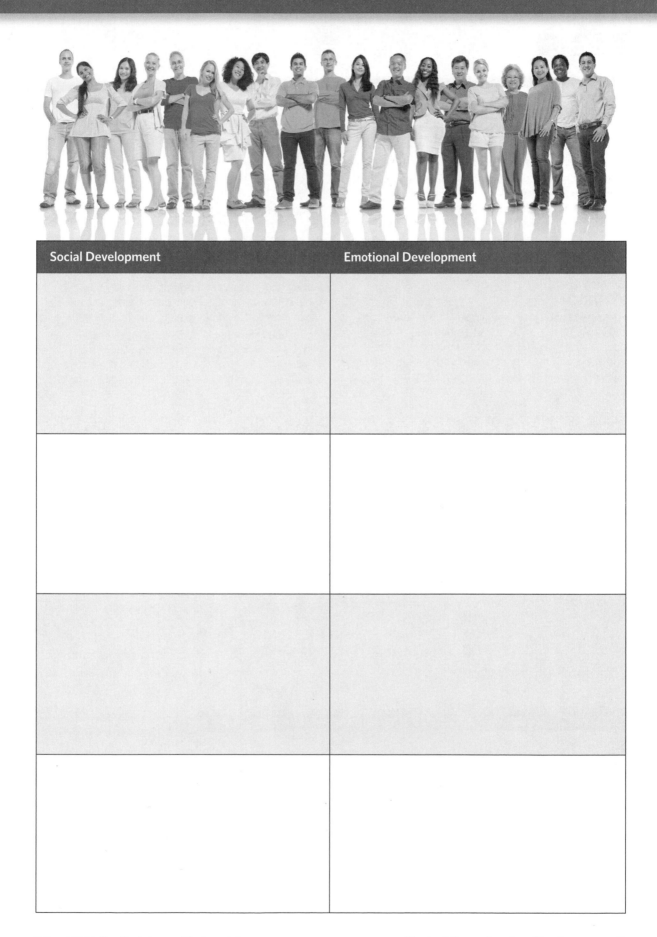

Social Development	Emotional Development

9.3 Motor Development Observation Lab

Within any group, there can be wide variation in developmental level and individual skill level. Teachers and coaches take these differences into account as each student matures and progresses to the next stage of development.

Name: _____

Date: _____

MISSION: Your teacher will arrange for you to observe Grade 9 or 10 students during a physical education class in which the students will be learning and/or practising a sport or a specific motor skill. *Note that all observations made during this exercise must remain strictly confidential and notes made must be respectful.*

You will work with a partner. At random and in agreement with your partner, select ten students in the class. Assign each of them a number. After you and your partner have selected your observation group of students and have agreed on your number identification system, both of you will go to opposite ends of the gym or playing field.

Independently of your partner, observe your group of ten students "in action" for 30 minutes. (Remember to perform your observations unobtrusively and without consulting your partner. You will compare notes with your partner at the end of the exercise.)

During your observation period, complete the table below as thoroughly as possible. Notes and observations should be detailed and neutral in tone.

When you return to class, discuss your observations with your partner. Did you agree on your observations of each student? Why or why not? What factors might explain some of the differences in the observations that you and your partner made?

Motor Development Observation Table

Date: _____

Grade level under observation: _____

Name of Instructor: _____

Individual (Numbered)	1	2	3	4	5	6	7	8	9	10
Sport or skill(s) being practised										
Estimated height of student (Tall/medium/short)										
Estimated weight of student (Heavy/average/underweight)										

Individual (Numbered)	1	2	3	4	5	6	7	8	9	10
Strength (Rate overall physical strength from 1 to 5—weak to strong)										
Balance (Rate overall balance from 1 to 5—very unstable to very stable)										
Coordination/agility (Rate overall coordination/ agility from 1 to 5—poorly coordinated/lacking in agility to very well coordinated/ extremely agile)										
Overall skill level (General rating of how well or how poorly student performed the sport or skill from 1 to 5—poor to excellent)										

General notes prior to comparing your observations with those of your partner.

9.4 Adapting Movement-Based Activities

Strong teachers and coaches understand the components of human growth and development and the various stages of the Long-Term Athlete Development model and adapt their training methods accordingly.

Name: _____

Date: _____

MISSION: Imagine you are the coach of a group of athletes whose developmental levels and chosen sports are indicated in the table below. Fill in as much information as possible about how you would modify the sport skills indicated based on each athlete's developmental level (i.e., LTAD stage).

In each case, indicate how you would address the four components of human development—physical, cognitive, emotional, and social—in adapting each physical action to match the specific developmental level. Keep in mind that you can modify equipment, basic rules of the sport, and several other factors in your attempts to match these activities to the appropriate developmental level. A sample entry is provided for you below.

Note: Assume that all of the athletes have "come through the ranks" in terms of the seven stages of the Long-Term Athlete Development (LTAD) model. In other words, a soccer player at Stage 2 (girls 6-8, boys 6-9) has already participated at Stage 1; a tennis player at Stage 3 (girls 8-11, boys 9-12) has already participated at Stages 1 and 2, and so on. One entry has been completed below to provide you with an example of how a movement-based activity can be adapted (i.e., modified) to suit a specific stage of development.

Sport Skill	LTAD Stage	Modification of Sport Skill
1. Hitting a baseball	Stage 1 (Active Start) (0-6 years)	Use a "tee," as a player of this age may have difficulty hitting a moving pitch. Use a light bat to allow for lack of physical strength. Work with the athlete to develop his or her swing without a ball, encouraging him or her to "visualize" contact repeatedly. Gradually introduce a slow-moving pitch with a larger ball for more advanced players. The social aspects of this skill may be challenging to develop as the skill is essentially individual.
2. Kicking a soccer ball	Stage 1 (Active Start) (0-6 years)	

3. **Heading a soccer ball**	Stage 2 (FUNdamentals) (girls 6-8, boys 6-9)	
4. **Passing a hockey puck**	Stage 2 (FUNdamentals) (girls 6-8, boys 6-9)	
5. **Performing a cartwheel in gymnastics**	Stage 3 (Learn to Train) (girls 8-11, boys 9-12)	
6. **Tossing a "spiral" pass in football**	Stage 3 (Learn to Train) (girls 8-11, boys 9-12)	
7. **Executing a jump shot in basketball**	Stage 4 (Train to Train) (girls 11-15, boys 12-16)	
8. **Executing a sand-trap shot in golf**	Stage 4 (girls 11-15, boys 12-16)	

Chapter 9 Quiz

The two sets of questions below will test your knowledge and broaden your understanding of the material covered in Chapter 9. Complete each set of questions according to your teacher's instructions.

Name: _____

Date: _____

Question Set 1: Physical Growth and Development

Multiple-Choice Questions

MISSION: Circle the letter beside the answer that you believe to be correct.

1. Human physical development encompasses
   (a) an individual's ability to interpret information
   (b) the ability to perform a wide range of tasks
   (c) relationships with peers, friends, and others
   (d) none of the above

2. Skeletal age
   (a) is indicated by the degree of ossification of bones
   (b) can be predicted according to chronological age
   (c) can be affected by diet, disease, and injury
   (d) all of the above

3. Which stage of human growth witnesses the most rapid physical development?
   (a) infancy/toddler
   (b) childhood
   (c) puberty/adolescence
   (d) adulthood

4. Significantly noticeable changes in physical appearance and body function in both sexes occur during
   (a) infancy
   (b) childhood/toddler
   (c) puberty/adolescence
   (d) adulthood

5. Which system secretes hormones to the body's various organs and tissues?
   (a) reproductive system
   (b) nervous system
   (c) endocrine system
   (d) lymphatic system

6. For youth aged 12-17, the Canadian Physical Activity Guidelines recommend at least
   (a) 60 minutes of physical activity per day
   (b) 30 minutes of physical activity per day
   (c) 120 minutes of physical activity per day
   (d) 90 minutes of physical activity per day

Short-Answer Questions

MISSION: Briefly answer the following questions in the space provided:

1. What are the differences between chronological, skeletal, and developmental age?

2. List the four key stages of human development.

3. List five factors affecting physical growth and development.

Essay Questions

MISSION: On a separate piece of paper, develop a 100-word response to the following questions.

1. Expand on the statement "Not all body parts and systems undergo physical change at the same rate."

2. Explain some implications of differing rates of physical development among adolescents.

3. From the perspective of the Canadian Society for Exercise Physiology (CSEP), what can we do throughout our lives to optimize our growth and development?

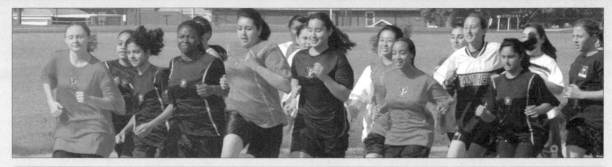

Courtesy of Tanya Winter

Question Set 2: Cognitive, Social, and Emotional Development and Activity Adaptation

Multiple-Choice Questions

MISSION: Circle the letter beside the answer that you believe to be correct.

1. The most widely accepted model of the stages of cognitive development was developed by
   (a) Jean Piaget
   (b) John Ratey
   (c) Jacob Sattelmeir
   (d) Henriette van Praag

2. The benefits of aerobic exercise include
   (a) neurogenesis (the birth of new neurons)
   (b) enhanced brain plasticity
   (c) prevention of brain tissue loss in older adults
   (d) all of the above

3. Children learn the give and take of social behaviour in general by interacting frequently with
   (a) teachers
   (b) friends
   (c) role models
   (d) parents or guardians

4. The Long-Term Athlete Development (LTAD) model takes into account a child's
   (a) chronological age
   (b) willingness to participate in physical activity
   (c) development and maturation
   (d) friendship network

5. A teacher or coach can identify a child as an early, average, or late maturer by using
   (a) peak height velocity charts
   (b) measurements of height, weight, and fat percentage
   (c) LTAD growth tracking tables
   (d) CSEP's Canadian Physical Activity Guidelines

6. It is important to design movement-based activities for children that match their physical, cognitive, social, and emotional abilities; such activities are described as
   (a) developmentally appropriate
   (b) socially beneficial
   (c) child-centred
   (d) character-building

Short-Answer Questions

MISSION: Briefly answer the following questions in the space provided:

1. What are the four stages of Jean Piaget's model of cognitive development?

2. List ways in which participation in sport and physical activity can enhance children's social development.

3. Why does Canadian Sport for Life promote the Long-Term Athlete Development (LTAD) model?

Essay Questions

MISSION: On a separate piece of paper, develop a 100-word response to the following questions.

1. Why is the modern field of child development indebted to Piaget's insights?

2. Discuss the role that sport participation and team membership can play in social interaction and relationship building.

3. Describe various ways to modify games, sports, or activities to match the developmental characteristics of children of varying ages, stages, and ability levels.

WORKSHEET

My Notes on Chapter 9

Use the space below to make notes on the questions on the facing page, to record any thoughts and ideas you have on this chapter, and to store study tips to help you prepare for tests and exams.

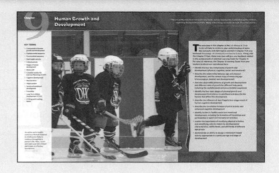

_____   _____
_____   _____
_____   _____
_____   _____
_____   _____
_____   _____
_____   _____
_____   _____
_____   _____
_____   _____
_____   _____
_____   _____
_____   _____
_____   _____
_____   _____
_____   _____
_____   _____
_____   _____
_____   _____
_____   _____
_____   _____
_____   _____
_____   _____

Chapter 9 Review (Student Textbook page 293)

Knowledge

1. Using a graphic organizer of your choice, identify and describe the four components of human growth and development. Then tell why it is important to look at each component to understand an individual's readiness to engage in physical activity and sport.

2. Develop a gender-specific timeline that illustrates in an appropriate and positive way the developmental stages experienced throughout the human lifespan along with various physical and sociocultural factors affecting development.

3. With a partner or in a small group, discuss various ways in which physical activity and/or sport can enhance healthy human social development.

4. List five positive effects of physical activity on cognitive functioning and development as demonstrated by researchers such as Dr. John Ratey.

5. How does Canadian Sport for Life's Long-Term Athlete Development Model strive to ensure a positive experience in physical activity and sport for everyone?

6. Describe three ways in which a complex skill can be modified or simplified to match the acquisition of the skill to the learner's ability level.

Thinking and Inquiry

7. Humans typically develop stability or balance skills first, followed by locomotor skills and then manipulation skills. Based upon this information, in performing what type of physical activities will pre-school children have the most success?

8. Physical activity that puts stress on your bones is vital for current and future bone health. Think back over the last seven days and list all of the physical activities that you did that would have helped to strengthen your bones. Based on that list, should you be doing more types of activities that will help benefit your bone development? What activities do you think you will continue to do as you get older to help ensure that your bones stay strong and healthy?

9. What are some potential benefits to educators and parents of understanding and applying Piaget's four-stage theory of cognitive development? Do you see any potential risks in applying Piaget's model? Explain why or why not.

10. How might you modify a volleyball game to accommodate the developmental stages and needs of a group of 9-to 12-year-olds?

11. If a friend tells you that a sport they used to enjoy now makes them feel exhausted and burned out, what might be one possible cause of this problem?

12. How could you modify a game of softball so that someone with a moderate visual impairment could participate?

13. What modifications could let a person who is hearing-impaired participate in a swimming race?

Communication

14. You have been asked to start up a new soccer league that is based on developmental age as opposed to chronological age. Write a brief proposal explaining how you might determine the developmental age of the players to ensure that the teams are equal.

15. Explain why positive social and emotional development early in life is extremely important for the development of friendships later in life.

16. What advice would you give a teacher or coach who wants to design a training and competition program for a child in early adolescence that will fit that child's level of readiness?

Application

17. Based on what you have learned in this chapter, think of three careers for which it is important to understand the characteristics of the different stages of human growth and development, and briefly explain your reasoning.

18. With a partner or in a small group, choose one of these age groups: pre-school (2 to 4); 5 to 6; 7 to 10; or 11 to 15. Select a physical activity, such as a yoga pose; a dance step; throwing, rolling, kicking, or bouncing a ball; striking a ball with a bat; running an obstacle course; hitting a badminton shuttle with a racquet; balancing on different parts of the body; or an activity of your choice. Design or modify the activity for your chosen age group so that it could be performed safely and successfully either in a gym, in a playground, or on a field. Present your movement-based activity design to the class for discussion. (Make sure your teacher approves it in advance.)

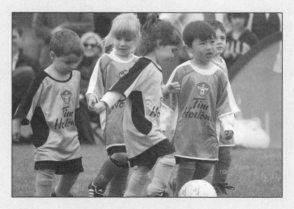

Three- and four-year-old children playing soccer in Oakville, Ontario, May 16, 2009. This is often the stage at which children first become introduced to organized sports and games. (CP Photo/Richard Buchan)

Motor Learning and Skill Acquisition

KEY TERMS

- Motor learning
- Stages of motor learning model
- Skill proficiency
- Phases of movement
- KP feedback
- KR feedback
- Sport psychology
- Ideal performance state
- Psychological skills training
- Canadian Sport for Life (CS4L)
- Long-Term Athlete Development (LTAD)
- Mental fitness
- Coaching styles
- Age-appropriate coaching strategies

Canada's Justine Colley, left, drives to the basket during a women's basketball match against Jamaica at the Pan American Games in Guadalajara, Mexico, in 2011.

AP Photo/Daniel Ochoa de Olza

The exercises in this chapter of the *Lab Manual & Study Guide* will help to reinforce your understanding of some key concepts and main topics covered in Chapter 10 of your textbook *Kinesiology: An Introduction to Exercise Science*. Along with the Chapter 10 Quiz, these exercises will give you feedback related to the achievement of selected Learning Goals for Chapter 10. For ease of reference, the Chapter 10 Learning Goals from your student textbook are reproduced here:

- describe three stages of human motor learning
- describe three stages of skill acquisition
- analyze movement skills in terms of three phases: preparation, execution, and follow-through
- describe the three categories of fundamental movement skills (FMS): stability, locomotor, and manipulation
- describe the role of feedback in skill acquisition
- explain the process of skill transferability in terms of the Long-Term Athlete Development (LTAD) model
- explain the basic principles of sport psychology, including why psychological factors are important for athletes and coaches in both training and competition
- describe psychological tools to help improve athletic performance, e.g., self-talk, imagery/visualization
- explain the relationship between mental fitness development and LTAD stages
- explain the influence of individual, environmental, and task-related constraints on skill acquisition and performance
- describe the crucial role of the coach in skill development
- identify the different approaches adopted by coaches
- explain how the concept of fair play relates to coaching
- describe how coaches adapt basic principles of skill development into age-appropriate coaching strategies for athletes of different ages and stages
- describe the contributions of prominent Canadians to sport

10.1 Motor Skills Observation Lab

When coaches and athletes break down the phases of a motor skill into key elements, they can look for ways to improve the execution of the skill. It is best to complete this exercise after you have studied Chapters 11-13 and 15.

Name: _____

Date: _____

(a) Hockey Skills Observation

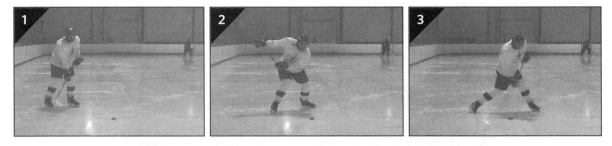

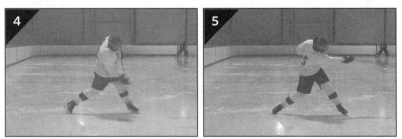

MISSION: Using the photographs above, identify the key elements of each phase of the skill and indicate training exercises that might result in improvement at each phase.

Phase	Key Elements of Phase	Training Exercises
1. Preliminary movements		
2. Back swing movements		
3. Force-producing movements		
4. Critical instant		
5. Follow-through		

(b) Soccer Skills Observation

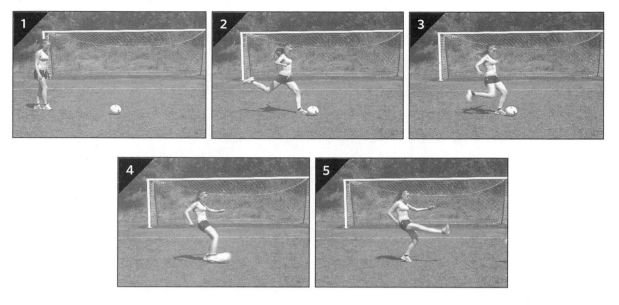

MISSION: Using the photographs above, identify the key elements of each phase of the skill and indicate training exercises that might result in improvement at each phase.

Phase	Key Elements of Phase	Training Exercises
1. Preliminary movements		
2. Back swing movements		
3. Force-producing movements		
4. Critical instant		
5. Follow-through		

(c) Golf Skills Observation

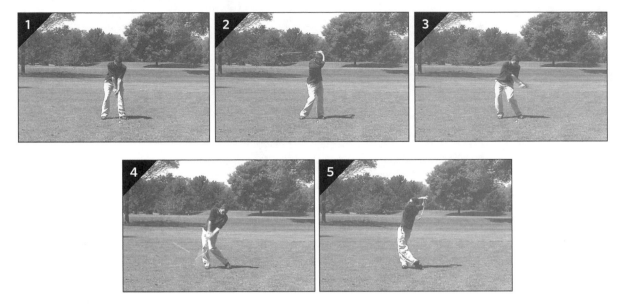

MISSION: Using the photographs above, identify the key elements of each phase of the skill and indicate training exercises that might result in improvement at each phase.

Phase	Key Elements of Phase	Training Exercises
1. Preliminary movements		
2. Back swing movements		
3. Force-producing movements		
4. Critical instant		
5. Follow-through		

(d) Tennis Skills Observation

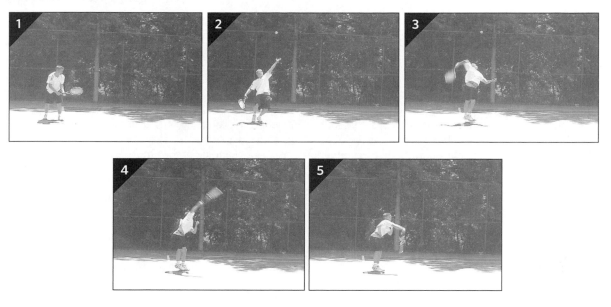

MISSION: Using the photographs above, identify the key elements of each phase of the skill and indicate training exercises that might result in improvement at each phase.

Phase	Key Elements of Phase	Training Exercises
1. Preliminary movements		
2. Back swing movements		
3. Force-producing movements		
4. Critical instant		
5. Follow-through		

10.2 Create a Sport Psychology Strategies Poster

Sport psychology is the study of the thought processes, feelings, and behaviour of people in the context of sports. Sport psychologists employ a wide range of techniques to help athletes stay focussed and achieve excellence.

Name: _____

Date: _____

MISSION: Your teacher will assign groups (with a maximum of five students per group). Each student in each group will choose a different sport psychology strategy to research, including, if they wish, a mental fitness actvity developed by Canadian Sport for Life as part of its Long-Term Athlete Development (LTAD) model. Examples of suitable strategies include:

- arousal/relaxation regulation
- neurofeedback training
- self-talk
- concentration enhancement and coping strategies
- motivation improvement
- imagery/visualization
- use of "cue words" to stay focussed
- mindfulness
- any other suitable topic approved by your teacher

In the table below, and on a separate sheet of paper if necessary, compile notes about the aspect of sport psychology that you have selected. Information should include a definition of the strategy, the basics of how it works to enhance performance, people who use it (athletes, coaches, and psychologists), and real-life examples of how it has been used to assist athletes.

Each student will have at least one class period to research their topic, and students can complete their research at home or at the library (perhaps using the template for an annotated bibliography on page 169).

After individual research is done, reconvene with your group to compile your findings into a poster. Each of the strategies should be represented in the poster.

Submit the poster to your teacher as a group (be sure to include the names of all group members). All group members should also hand in their individual research notes for evaluation.

Research Areas	Initial Research Notes
Description of selected topic or strategy	
How the strategy tends to be used	
Famous coaches/athletes/ psychologists who use the strategy	
When was the strategy first used?	
How does the strategy work?	

Sport Psychology—Annotated Bibliography

An annotated bibliography is a brief synopsis of a book or journal article that is pertinent to a given research topic of interest. It follows a particular style and format, as shown below.

MISSION: Select a topic related to sport psychology and in the table below, annotate three different articles or books that discuss your chosen topic. Keep a hard copy of the article or book for reference, or store material in an online folder. A sample entry is provided below.

Author(s), Title of Book or Article, Source	Summary of Findings
Hassell, Kristina, Catherine M. Sabinston, and Gordon A. Bloom (McGill University, Canada, October-December 2010). Exploring the multiple dimensions of social support among elite female adolescent swimmers. *International Journal of Sport Psychology*, 41 (4), 340–359.	This study explored multiple dimensions of social support of nine elite female adolescent swimmers. Results highlighted the importance of the structural, functional, and perceptual social support dimensions on athletes' experiences in elite swimming in relation to their coaches, parents, and peers. Coaches were an important provider of almost every aspect of social support. Teammates provided a sense of affiliation and shared experience that was described as the most positive aspect of their swimming involvement.
1.	
2.	
3.	

WORKSHEET

10.3 Coaching Styles

Coaches at all levels of sport adopt a wide range of coaching styles and methods when working with athletes. A coach's approach to training and competition has a huge impact on how well a team or an athlete performs.

Name: _____

Date: _____

MISSION: Select one of the following coaches and do some research to answer the questions that follow.

- ✔ Amélie Mauresmo
- ✔ Robin McKeever
- ✔ Melissa Basilio
- ✔ John Herdman

- ✔ Pat Summitt
- ✔ Dwayne Casey
- ✔ Randy Carlyle
- ✔ Kathy Shields

- ✔ Ted Nolan
- ✔ Shawnee Harle
- ✔ Any other coach approved by your teacher

Questions

1. For what sport is this coach best known? _____

2. Which one of the coaching styles outlined in your textbook does she or he demonstrate?

   _____

3. Is this coach best described as autocratic or democratic?

   _____

4. How does this coach motivate athletes? Provide examples from actual competitions to support your answer.

   _____

   _____

5. Based on the discussion in the textbook about fair play and the ethical behaviour of coaches, would you say that this coach deals with matters in a fair and ethical manner? Again, give examples to justify your answers.

   _____

   _____

6. Indicate one instance in which this coach applied a superior knowledge of strategies or tactics to the benefit of his or her athlete(s) in a competitive situation.

   _____

7. If you were an athlete, would you like to work with the coach you selected? Why, or why not?

   _____

8. If you were a coach, would you attempt to emulate the coach you have chosen? Why, or why not?

   _____

A Comparison of Coaching Styles

A coach's style is heavily influenced by the age and developmental level of their athletes. Coaches use different, age-appropriate coaching strategies, based on an understanding of the Long-Term Athlete Development (LTAD) model, to elicit the best performances from athletes or teams.

MISSION: Select two coaches in your school and/or community and observe their coaching styles during a practice session. As you observe the two practice sessions one after the other, complete the following chart by placing a check mark in the box beside that specific coaching style each time you observe behaviours associated with that style exhibited by the coach. Remember to obtain approval from your teacher and from each coach that you would like to observe before you begin this exercise.

Coaches' Names	_____	_____
Sport	_____	_____
LTAD level of athlete(s)	_____	_____

Coaching Style	Definition	Coach 1	Coach 2
Authoritarian			
Business-like			
"Nice guy/gal"			
Intense			
"Easy-going"			

WORKSHEET

Chapter 10 Quiz

The two sets of questions below will test your knowledge and broaden your understanding of the material covered in Chapter 10. Complete each set of questions according to your teacher's instructions.

Name: _____

Date: _____

Question Set 1: Motor Learning and Skill Acquisition

Multiple-Choice Questions

MISSION: Circle the letter beside the answer that you believe to be correct.

1. The process through which a person develops the ability to perform and refine a task or skill is called
   (a) physical development
   (b) psychological development
   (c) rudimentary learning
   (d) motor learning

2. The root of any motor activity lies in the
   (a) musculoskeletal system
   (b) sensory and nervous systems
   (c) decision mechanism
   (d) effector mechanism

3. What is the name given to the body's "mechanism" that coordinates the mental commands and physical responses needed to produce movement?
   (a) effector
   (b) decision
   (c) memory
   (d) perceptual

4. The earliest and still most widely used approach to understanding how humans acquire skills is the
   (a) Long-Term Athlete Development Model
   (b) stages of motor learning model
   (c) Newell's Model of Constraints
   (d) Gallahue and Donnelly's five-step approach to KP feedback

5. The three basic categories of fundamental movement skills are
   (a) stability, flexibility, and manipulation
   (b) stability, locomotion, and manipulation
   (c) stability, rotation, and manipulation
   (d) stability, coordination, and manipulation

6. The ability to apply skills learned in the context of improving performance in one activity to a different activity is called
   (a) skill versatility
   (b) skill specialization
   (c) skill transferability
   (d) skill consolidation

Short-Answer Questions

MISSION: Briefly answer the following questions in the space provided:

1. For a learner to improve skill performance, what type of feedback is most effective?

2. Into which three components or phases of movement can a skill be broken down?

3. Why is skill transferability important when learning new motor skills?

Essay Questions

MISSION: On a separate piece of paper, develop a 100-word response to the following questions.

1. Apply the stages of learning model developed by Fitts and Posner in describing how someone develops proficiency in learning to throw a ball.

2. Explain the important role of feedback in skill acquisition and performance. Distinguish between two categories of feedback.

3. Explain how participation in well-structured physical activities that develop fundamental movement skills helps children develop physical literacy over the long term.

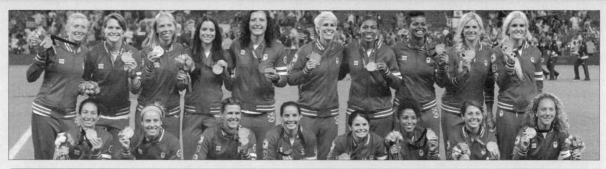

CP Photo/Frank Gunn

Question Set 2: Sport Psychology and the Important Role of Coaching in Skill Acquisition

Multiple-Choice Questions

MISSION: Circle the letter beside the answer that you believe to be correct.

1. The role of sports psychologist includes
   (a) teaching athletes how to block out crowd noise
   (b) working with coaches and athletes to improve motivation
   (c) helping competitors to avoid feelings of anxiety that inhibit performance
   (d) all of the above

2. In the mind of an athlete, a sense of effortlessness and the feeling that time has "stood still" describes
   (a) "the zone"
   (b) an ideal performance state
   (c) choking
   (d) both (a) and (b) are correct

3. Breathing control exercises, progressive relaxation exercises, meditation, and imagery all help control
   (a) arousal
   (b) relaxation
   (c) anxiety
   (d) concentration

4. Techniques for improving an athlete's concentration include
   (a) positive self-talk
   (b) neurofeedback training
   (c) use of cue words
   (d) all of the above

5. Skills that emphasize attitude, positive focus, imagination, effort, and fun are known as
   (a) visualization strategies
   (b) coping strategies
   (c) motivational skills
   (d) mental fitness skills

6. Successful coaches continuously seek to
   (a) help athletes develop relaxation, imagery, concentration and coping skills
   (b) remain alert to symptoms of burnout, anxiety, or depression in their athletes
   (c) improve relationships with their athletes
   (d) all of the above

Short-Answer Questions

MISSION: Briefly answer the following questions in the space provided:

1. Define motivation in sport and list several key factors that are associated with motivation.

2. Define "coaching styles" and identify five types of coaching styles.

3. What are some important points to keep in mind when coaches work with children in sports?

Essay Questions

MISSION: On a separate piece of paper, develop a 100-word response to the following questions.

1. Research any three famous athletes who have benefitted from using mental fitness strategies, and explain how they used sport psychology to their advantage.

2. Imagine you are a coach who has been hired to work with a top-level athlete who has recently been feeling unmotivated or "burned out." Outline the steps you would take in working with the athlete to try to overcome this impediment to his or her performance.

WORKSHEET

My Notes on Chapter 10

Use the space below to make notes on the
questions on the facing page, to record any
thoughts and ideas you have on this chapter,
and to store study tips to help you prepare for
tests and exams.

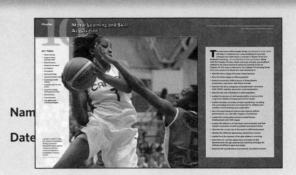

Name

Date

_____

_____

_____

_____

_____

_____

_____

_____

_____

_____

_____

_____

_____

_____

_____

_____

_____

_____

_____

_____

_____

_____

Chapter 10 Review (Student Textbook page 317)

Knowledge

1. In a table, identify and describe what makes the cognitive, associative, and autonomous stages of motor learning unique from each other.

2. Choose a motor skill such as doing a push-up or a biceps curl, rolling a ball, doing a stride jump or a long jump, or any other skill that you have performed or have observed a peer perform. Make a simple labelled sketch showing someone performing the skill during each of the three stages of skill acquisition.

3. Using a graphic organizer of your choice, place each of these fundamental movement skills into the appropriate skill category (i.e., stability, locomotor, or manipulation): (a) throwing, (b) kicking, (c) skipping, (d) galloping, (e) stork stand, (f) log roll, (g) dribbling a ball with your hands, (h) striking a ball with a bat, (i) running, and (j) skating.

4. Identify the characteristics of an athlete who is in an ideal performance state (in "the zone").

5. Describe four specific tools that sport psychologists and athletes apply in the course of "psychological skills training" (PST) to improve athletic performance, and state why each tool has proven successful.

6. "There is a lot more to coaching than an ability to impart knowledge of rules and basic skills." Expand on this statement based on what you have learned about effective coaching styles and aptitudes.

Thinking and Inquiry

7. The following are various components of hopping. Identify in which phase of the hopping skill (i.e., preparation, execution, or follow-through) each component belongs: • Swing leg swings forward and upward to produce thrust • Push off balls of feet• Pendulum action of swing leg• Body upright, look forward, arms bent at side at 90 degrees• Landing softly on balls of feet, slight ankle and knee flexion• Rhythmical swing of arms on take-off

8. As one of your peers throws a ball, you notice that he or she continually throws the ball to the right of the intended target. What might be some reasons for this behaviour and what feedback could you provide to help the person improve their throwing skill?

9. In a group or with a partner, analyze the benefits of organizing mental fitness activities into pre-performance, performance, and post-performance phases, as in the Long-Term Athlete Development Model.

10. If you have just begun coaching an athlete who typically experiences a great deal of anxiety prior to a competitive event, what kind of guidance, tools, and advice could you provide to help the individual gain control of negative emotions?

11. Think of the last time you practised a motor skill during a game, sport, physical education class, or recreational activity. Describe the constraints that either limited or facilitated your performance.

Communication

12. Fundamental movement skills form the foundation for more complex and sport-specific skills. Choose one fundamental movement skill and create a poster, slideshow , or other medium demonstrating how proficiency in this skill can be transferred to proficiency in five more complex and sport-specific skills.

13. Conduct research to find one or more examples of an athlete who demonstrates how developing and refining mental fitness skills and attributes can help enhance performance and mental well-being. Present your findings to the class in a brief report.

Application

14. Identify a skill that you are unable to perform. Examples might include juggling three tennis balls, performing a head stand, or executing a particular dance step. Do some research to learn how to perform this skill. Based on the descriptions for each stage of motor learning, try to progress from the cognitive stage to the associative stage of the skill.

15. Identify a physical activity or sport that you enjoy. Identify as many factors as possible that motivate you to participate in this activity. What strategies do you employ to prevent boredom from setting in?

16. Write out brief descriptions of the stages involved in performing an overhand throw. Then use the proper technique to throw a ball back and forth with a partner using your non-dominant hand. Describe what you notice about how a skill that is initially performed at the cognitive stage (i.e., using your non-dominant hand) improves when you learn how it is performed at either the associative or autonomous stage (i.e., using the dominant hand).

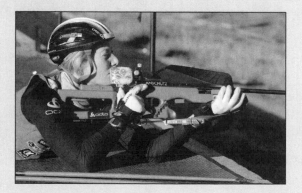

Biathletes who undergo neurofeedback training learn how to control their physiological reactions to stress. This sense of control leads to a state of regulation over mind and body that can result in enhanced performance. (CP Photo/ Larry MacDougal)

Biomechanical Theory and Concepts

KEY TERMS

- Biomechanics
- Force
- Newton's laws of motion
- Inertia
- Acceleration
- Linear (or translational) motion
- Angular (or rotational) motion
- Torque
- Ergonomics

Canadian snowboarder Michael Lambert makes his way down the men's parallel slalom during qualification runs for the 2014 Winter Olympics in Sochi, Russia.

John Lehmann/The Globe and Mail

The exercises in this chapter of the *Lab Manual & Study Guide* will help to reinforce your understanding of some key concepts and main topics covered in Chapter 11 of your textbook *Kinesiology: An Introduction to Exercise Science*. Along with the Chapter 11 Quiz, these exercises will give you feedback related to the achievement of selected Learning Goals for Chapter 11. For ease of reference, the Chapter 11 Learning Goals from your student textbook are reproduced here:

- define the term "biomechanics" and explain its application to understanding proficiency of human movement

- explain biomechanical theory and concepts as they relate to the study of human movement

- differentiate between internal and external forces

- describe the contributions of Sir Isaac Newton to the field of physics and biomechanics

- explain Newton's three laws of motion in relation to stationary and moving objects

- define three types of levers and identify lever systems in the human body and in sport and physical activity

- differentiate between linear motion, rotational motion, and general motion

- differentiate between centric and eccentric (off-centre) forces

- explain what determines which type of motion occurs

- describe some real-world applications of knowledge of biomechanics, including the development of prosthetics and other innovative designs related to sport

- identify some careers related to biomechanics

John Lehmann/The Globe and Mail

WORKSHEET

11.1 Types of Forces and Newton's Laws

All of our bodily movements can be understood in the context of external and internal forces and Newton's three universal laws of motion. Biomechanics can be defined as the application of Newton's laws to human movement.

Name: _____

Date: _____

(A) Fill in the Blanks

MISSION: Fill in the correct term from those provided here. Some terms may be used more than once.

minimize imbalance acceleration internal direction inertia external equilibrium magnitude maximize

1. A force is any influence, internal or external, that causes an object or a body to undergo movement, or a change in movement or _____.

2. Because forces have both _____ and direction, they are known as vector quantities.

3. All observed movement results from a(n) _____ of forces acting on a body.

4. In the study of human motion, there could be any number of forces, both _____ and _____, acting at any given time and in any given situation.

5. To move proficiently or help others do the same, we need to understand how to _____ the benefits of forces and at the same time _____ their potential harmful effects, such as injuries.

6. A swimmer encounters water resistance while performing a front crawl in a pool. Water resistance is an example of a(n) _____ force.

7. In biomechanics, the human body is regarded as a system and any force exerted by one part of the body on another, for example, when a muscle contracts to move a joint, is a(n) _____ force.

8. The property of matter that causes an object or body to resist any changes in motion is known as _____.

9. When two objects exert equal and opposite forces against each other such that the sum of the forces when added together equals zero, the two objects are said to be in a state of _____ and no motion is observed.

10. The rate at which the velocity of an object changes over time is known as _____.

(B) True or False?

MISSION: Circle whether each statement is True (T) or False (F).

1. Newton's first law of motion, also known as the law of inertia, applies only when an object is in a stationary position and not when an object is in a state of motion. T/F

2. The more mass an object has, the greater its inertia and the more effort it will take to cause the object to move or to stop moving. T/F

3. According to Newton's second law of motion, if a small force is applied to an object, the object will experience a large change in its velocity (the rate at which it is moving). T/F

4. The acceleration experienced by a ping pong ball and a tennis ball to which a force of equal magnitude is applied will differ because the two objects differ in volume. T/F

5. When a basketball rests motionless on a gymnasium floor, the floor exerts an unequal and opposite force upward on the basketball. T/F

6. When a speedskater pushes off at the start of a race, the surface of the ice exerts a force that is equal and opposite in magnitude to the force applied by the skater. T/F

(C) Newton's Three Laws of Motion

MISSION: In the table below, write Newton's three laws of motion in the first column and an example of a physical activity or sport that demonstrates each law in the second column. In the third column, write a brief rationale explaining how each physical activity or sport demonstrates that particular law of motion.

Newton's Law	Physical Activity or Sport	Rationale
The First Law of Motion (Inertia):		
The Second Law of Motion (Acceleration):		
The Third Law of Motion (Reaction):		

WORKSHEET

11.2 Levers in the Human Body

A lever in the human body consists of a rigid structure (e.g., a long bone) that rotates about a fixed point or fulcrum (a joint). The distances of the load and the effort from the fulcrum affect the type of movement that takes place.

Name: _____

Date: _____

(A) Types of Levers

MISSION: Complete the information below for each class of lever. Draw a diagram in each box provided.

First Class Lever

The applied force or effort (E) and the load or resistance (R) are located on opposite sides of the fulcrum (F). Provides a force advantage or a speed advantage, depending on where the fulcrum is located.

Diagram of a first class lever:

F = Fulcrum

E = Effort (or Force)

R = Resistance

Everyday example of a first class lever: _____

Example of a first class lever in the human body: _____

Second Class Lever

The resistance or load (R) is between the fulcrum and the applied force or effort (E). Provides a force advantage.

Diagram of a second class lever:

F = Fulcrum

E = Effort (or Force)

R = Resistance

Everyday example of a second class lever: _____

Example of a second class lever in the human body: _____

Third Class Lever

The applied force or effort (E) is located between the fulcrum (F) and the load or resistance (R). Tends to provide a speed advantage rather than a force advantage.

Diagram of a third class lever:

F = Fulcrum

E = Effort (or Force)

R = Resistance

Everyday example of a third class lever: _____

Example of a third class lever in the human body: _____

(B) Levers and Human Movement

MISSION: Each of the bodily movements listed below involves the action of a lever. For each movement, use words or sketches to identify the relative positions of the effort force (E), the fulcrum (F), and the resistance or load (R). In the first column, identify which class of lever is involved in each movement.

Movement	Effort Force (E)	Fulcrum / Axis (F)	Resistance (R)
Knee extension Class of lever: _____			
Shoulder adduction Class of lever: _____			
Elbow extension Class of lever: _____			
Hip extension Class of lever: _____			
Scapular elevation Class of lever: _____			

WORKSHEET

11.3 Types of Motion

Biomechanists classify the motion of a body or an object as predominantly either "linear" or "angular." Human movement that is a combination of both linear and angular components is referred to as "general motion."

Name: _____

Date: _____

(A) Distinguishing Types of Motion

MISSION: Complete the table below to demonstrate your understanding of the ways in which biomechanists categorize types of motion.

Classify each movement or action listed in the table as involving predominantly linear motion or predominantly rotational motion (check one or the other). Provide a brief rationale for each of your classifications in the appropriate cells of the table.

Movement or Action		Rationale
1. A diver twists in the air after jumping off a diving board. *Primarily:* □ Linear □ Angular		
2. A ski jumper slides down a run in a crouched position. *Primarily:* □ Linear □ Angular		
3. A ballet dancer performs a pirouette. *Primarily:* □ Linear □ Angular		
4. A basketball player pivots on one foot to make a pass. *Primarily:* □ Linear □ Angular		
5. A bowler approaches the foul line prior to rolling the ball. *Primarily:* □ Linear □ Angular		
6. A four-man bobsled team begins its slide down a track. *Primarily:* □ Linear □ Angular		

(B) Understanding Rotational Motion

MISSION: Answer the questions below to demonstrate your understanding of rotational motion and the kind of force that produces rotational motion.

Describe three different ways in which human physical activities can involve rotational (or angular) motion. You can give some examples from your own experience of these three kinds of rotational motion.

1. _____

   _____

   _____

2. _____

   _____

   _____

3. _____

   _____

   _____

4. Which characteristic of a force determines whether or not the object to which the force is applied will undergo rotational motion? Draw two simple labelled diagrams in the spaces below to support your answer.

   _____

   _____

   _____

Chapter 11 Quiz

The two sets of questions below will test your knowledge and broaden your understanding of the material covered in Chapter 11. Complete each set of questions according to your teacher's instructions.

Name: _____

Date: _____

Question Set 1: Newton's Laws of Motion and Levers in the Human Body

Multiple-Choice Questions

MISSION: Circle the letter beside the answer that you believe to be correct.

1. An example of Isaac Newton's first law of motion (inertia) would be:
   (a) a basketball resting motionless on the floor
   (b) a rock travelling endlessly into outer space
   (c) a bowling ball rolling evenly down a lane
   (d) all of the above

2. According to Newton's second law of motion (acceleration), a force applied to an object causes an acceleration of that object of a magnitude that is
   (a) unrelated to the object's mass
   (b) inversely proportional to the object's mass
   (c) the same as the object's mass
   (d) directly proportional to the force itself

3. According to Newton's second law of motion (stated as $F = ma$), the acceleration of a 0.33 kg tennis ball when a force of 10 N is applied to it will be
   (a) 3.3 m/s^2
   (b) 33.3 m/s^2
   (c) 333.3 ms^2
   (d) 3333.3 ms^2

4. An example of Newton's third law of motion (action-reaction) would be
   (a) a diver pushing off a diving platform
   (b) a basketball player jumping up to take a shot
   (c) a kettlebell resting on a gymnasium floor
   (d) all of the above

5. A mechanical device where the force is applied between the fulcrum and the load is a
   (a) first-class lever
   (b) second-class lever
   (c) third-class lever
   (d) none of the above

6. Plantarflexion is an example of a
   (a) first-class lever
   (b) second-class lever
   (c) third-class lever
   (d) none of the above

Short-Answer Questions

MISSION: Briefly answer the following questions in the space provided:

1. Define the term "biomechanics."

2. What is meant by the phrase "movement proficiency"?

3. Name the four components of a lever, list each type of lever, with an example, and state what general advantage each type of lever provides.

Essay Questions

MISSION: On a separate piece of paper, develop a 100-word response to the following questions.

1. Explain, with examples, how external and internal forces can either help or hinder movement, depending on the context.

2. Discuss whether you think understanding Newton's laws of motion is essential in understanding human movement and sport.

3. Identify and describe a bone-muscle-joint configuration that represents a third-class lever. Sketch this configuration and label the fulcrum, the load, and the effort.

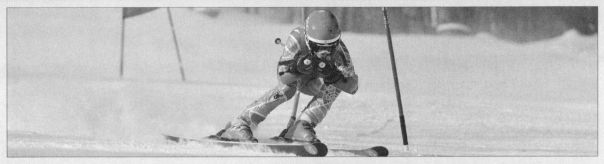

Courtesy of Zach Temertzoglou

Question Set 2: Types of Motion and Applied Biomechanics

Multiple-Choice Questions

MISSION: Circle the letter beside the answer that you believe to be correct.

1. Motion that takes place when a body or its collective parts moves the same distance in the same direction in the same amount of time is known as
   (a) rectilinear motion
   (b) translational motion
   (c) linear motion
   (d) all of the above

2. The linear motion of humans is generally a result of the interaction of
   (a) a combination of forces
   (b) a combination of diagonal movements
   (c) a combination of forward movements
   (d) none of the above

3. Generally, a force acting through the centre of an object or body will cause the object or body to
   (a) rotate clockwise
   (b) rotate counterclockwise
   (c) rotate sideways
   (d) move in a straight line

4. The turning effect produced by an eccentric force applied to a body at some distance from an axis of rotation is known as
   (a) velocity
   (b) angular motion
   (c) the resultant force
   (d) torque

5. Human movement is usually a combination of linear and rotational motion and is called
   (a) resultant motion
   (b) general motion
   (c) accelerated motion
   (d) projectile motion

6. Ergonomists match these human characteristics to specific activities.
   (a) cognitive and psychological
   (b) anatomical, physiological, and biomechanical
   (c) musculoskeletal and neurological
   (d) none of the above

Short-Answer Questions

MISSION: Briefly answer the following questions in the space provided:

1. List three different ways in which human physical activity can involve rotational or angular motion.

2. How can linear movements such as walking and running involve angular motion as well?

3. Distinguish between a centric and an eccentric force. What is the result of each type of force?

Essay Questions

MISSION: On a separate piece of paper, develop a 100-word response to the following questions.

1. Explain what determines which type of motion occurs when a force is applied to a stationary object or body.

2. Define the term "ergonomics" and give examples of everyday devices to which ergonomic thinking has been applied.

3. Biomechanics is an "applied science." What are some areas in which biomechanics would have practical uses? Give several examples of career paths related to biomechanics.

WORKSHEET

My Notes on Chapter 11

Use the space below to make notes on the questions on the facing page, to record any thoughts and ideas you have on this chapter, and to store study tips to help you prepare for tests and exams.

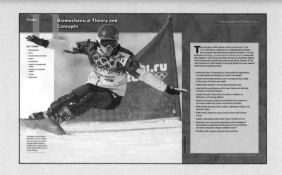

Chapter 11 Review (Student Textbook page 335)

Knowledge

1. Define the term "biomechanics" and state several purposes driving the work that biomechanists do.

2. Define the terms "force," "internal force," and "external force" and give one example for each term. What is the unit of measurement of a force?

3. There are three classes of levers. Select and describe or sketch three real-life examples that can help you remember the relative positioning of the fulcrum, the point of application of the effort force, and the load (or resistance) in each class of lever.

4. Linear motion, also called translational motion, is motion in a straight line. What are three defining characteristics of linear motion?

5. Give three examples of linear motion in the context of (a) human movement in sports; and (b) human movement during everyday activities.

6. Angular (rotational) motion is motion that takes place about an axis. Give three examples of angular motion in the context of (a) a sport; and (b) joint movements in the human body. For each example, identify the axis of rotation.

7. List three ways in which both individuals and society can benefit from applied knowledge of biomechanics.

Thinking and Inquiry

8. Create a mnemonic (an acronym or a memorable phrase) that can help you understand and recall each of Newton's three laws of motion.

9. Which class of lever is most commonly found in the human body, and why do you think this is the case? Give some examples to support your thinking.

10. More often than not, human movement is a result of the interaction of a combination of forces. Think of one example (other than the forward movement of a football lineman) for which a biomechanist could use basic trigonometry to compute a resultant force causing linear motion.

11. Use a Venn diagram to compare and contrast linear motion and angular (rotational) motion.

12. Give three examples of general motion other than the ones provided in your text.

Communication

13. Work in a small group to find and cut out images in newspapers or magazines that depict Newton's laws of motion in real-life settings. Arrange the images into a collage under the headings "Inertia," "Acceleration," and "Action-Reaction."

14. Draw labelled sketches showing examples of human joint arrangements that represent each class of lever.

15. Make a brief presentation in class in which you use everyday objects to show the two ways in which the introduction of a force can disturb equilibrium (by causing an imbalance in forces), thus causing a change in the motion of an object.

16. Many movements in sport involve the application of an eccentric or "off-centre" force that results in rotation about an axis. Using stick figure drawings, identify the point of application of a force and the axis of rotation in each of the following examples: (a) a football tackle, (b) a judo throw, and c) a biceps curl.

Application

17. Choose a motor skill, demonstrate the skill to a classmate or a friend, and explain how that skill involves a combination of all of Newton's laws of motion more or less at the same time.

18. Using brooms, hockey sticks, or similar objects, demonstrate the three classes of levers. For each class of lever, identify the relative positions of the fulcrum, the point of application of the effort force, and the load (resistance). Explain the type of advantage that each class of lever provides.

19. Perform a specific physical movement (or observe someone performing a movement), for example, a slap shot, a tennis serve, walking, or running. Identify the linear components of the movement. Which concepts could you apply to separate out these components for measurement and analysis?

20. Biomechanical research conducted by universities or private companies often seeks to understand and improve everyday physical movements. If you could participate in a research project, which one would you choose, and why?

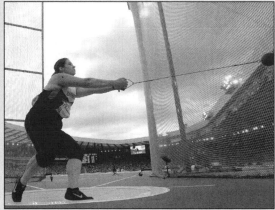

Canada's Sultana Frizell, from Perth, Ontario, generated powerful rotational forces in executing the movements that won her the gold medal in the women's hammer throw competition at the 2014 Commonwealth Games in Glasgow, Scotland. (AP Photo/Frank Augstein)

The Seven Principles of Biomechanics

KEY TERMS

- Statics
- Dynamics
- Stability
- Balance
- Mass
- Centre of mass
- Base of support
- Position of the centre of mass
- Joint range of motion
- Momentum
- Velocity
- Impulse
- Fosbury Flop
- Impulse-momentum relationship
- Torque
- Angle of insertion
- Angular momentum
- Angular velocity
- Moment of inertia
- Law of conservation of momentum

Devon Kershaw of Sudbury (front) and Alex Harvey (right) of St-Fereol-les-Neiges, Québec, in the 50 km cross-country race at the Canadian championship in 2012. Both athletes crossed the finish line together to win the race.

CP Photo/Jacques Boissinot

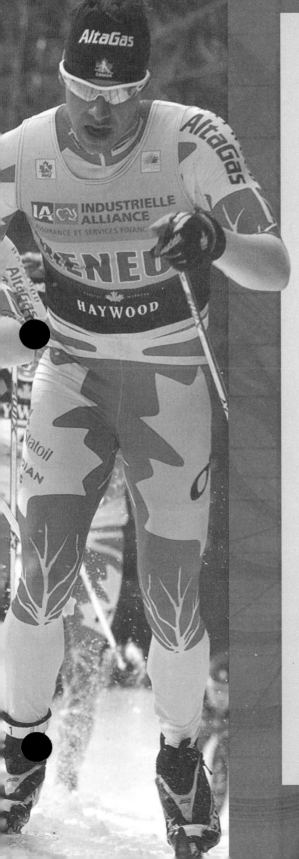

The exercises in this chapter of the *Lab Manual & Study Guide* will help to reinforce your understanding of some key concepts and main topics covered in Chapter 12 of your textbook *Kinesiology: An Introduction to Exercise Science*. Along with the Chapter 12 Quiz, these exercises will give you feedback related to the achievement of selected Learning Goals for Chapter 12. For ease of reference, the Chapter 12 Learning Goals from your student textbook are reproduced here:

- differentiate between static and dynamic systems in terms of human movement patterns

- demonstrate an understanding of human movement patterns as a product of multiple internal and external forces

- demonstrate an understanding of the biomechanical principle related to stability

- demonstrate an understanding of the two biomechanical principles related to maximum effort (i.e., production of maximum force; sequencing of joint rotation)

- demonstrate an understanding of the two biomechanical principles related to linear motion (i.e., the impulse-momentum relationship; the direction of the applied force)

- demonstrate an understanding of the two biomechanical principles related to angular motion (i.e., the effect of a force acting at some distance from an axis; the conservation of angular momentum)

- describe various applications of biomechanical principles related to skill improvement and enhanced athletic performance

WORKSHEET

12.1 The Seven Principles of Biomechanics: Anchor Chart

You can begin to understand movement dynamics and biomechanical analysis through the seven biomechanical principles set forth by the Coaching Association of Canada's National Coaching Certification Program (NCCP).

Name: _____

Date: _____

MISSION: As you read through Chapter 12 in your textbook, demonstrate your understanding of the seven principles of biomechanics by completing the table below as you progress through the chapter.

- The biomechanical principle is stated for you in the first column of the table.
- In the second column, rewrite the principle in your own words. If you like, create a simple sketch or diagram to help you understand each principle.
- In the third column, describe, in point form, one or more activity-specific or sport-specific example(s) of the principle in action.

The Seven Principles of Biomechanics: Anchor Chart for Reference and Review		
Biomechanical Principle	**Restated In Your Own Words**	**Example(s) of Principle in Action**
Principle 1: Stability The greater the mass, the lower the centre of mass to the base of support, the larger the base of support, and the closer the centre of mass is positioned to the base of support, the more stability increases.		
Principle 2: Production of Maximum Force The production of maximum force requires the use of all possible joint movements that contribute to the task's objective.		
Principle 3: Production of Maximum Velocity The production of maximum velocity requires the use of joints in order—from largest to smallest.		

Principle 4: The Impulse-Momentum Relationship		
The greater the applied impulse, the greater the increase in velocity.		
Principle 5: Direction of Force Application Movement usually occurs in the direction opposite that of the applied force.		
Principle 6: Production of Angular Motion (Torque) Angular motion is produced by the application of a force acting at some distance from an axis; that is, by torque.		
Principle 7: Conservation of Angular Momentum Angular momentum is constant when an individual or object is free in the air.		

12.2 Principle 1: Stability

The ability to maintain one's balance is crucial in almost every physical activity or sport. Biomechanical principle 1 applies whether you are on a sidewalk, a skateboard, a bike, a balance beam, or a football field.

Name: _____

Date: _____

MISSION 1: Assume each of the following positions and determine their relative stability by having your partner push you *gently and continuously* with two hands on the anterior part of your shoulders to try to upset your balance. Then, answer the questions that follow.

   (a) standing upright on one foot

   (b) standing upright on two feet, feet together

   (c) standing upright on two feet, feet shoulder width apart

   (d) standing upright on two feet with weight displaced forward, leaning with both hands on a metre stick placed about two-thirds of a metre in front of you (like a cane held with both hands)

   (e) standing upright on two feet with weight displaced forward, leaning on a chair

   (f) standing upright on two feet, feet placed one foot in front of the other about one metre apart

1. Which position is the most stable, relatively speaking? Explain your observations.

   _____

   _____

   _____

   _____

   _____

   _____

   _____

2. Which position is the least stable, relatively speaking? Explain your observations.

   _____

   _____

   _____

   _____

   _____

   _____

   _____

MISSION 2: Repeat positions (a) to (f) on the previous page, but this time have your partner push you *gently* from the lateral side of your shoulder when you assume each position.

Answer the following questions:

1. Which position is the most stable, relative to the other positions? Explain your observations.

   _____

   _____

   _____

   _____

   _____

2. Which position is the least stable, relative to the other positions? Explain your observations.

   _____

   _____

   _____

   _____

   _____

3. Describe three specific examples in sport where the base of support and stability (or a lack of stability) can benefit performance.

   (a) _____

   (b) _____

   (c) _____

MISSION 3: Stand up, bend from the waist, and touch your toes without bending your knees. Now, repeat these actions, but this time stand with your gluteus maximus and both of your calcaneous touching the wall. What result do you observe?

Why do you think this is the case? (Relate your observations to the centre of gravity, the line of gravity, and the base of support.)

_____

_____

_____

_____

_____

_____

_____

12.3 Principles 2 and 3: Maximum Effort

When participating in many activities and sports, we must exert maximum effort to accomplish a specific task—for example, lifting a heavy object, running as far as possible, or striking a ball or other object during a game.

Name: _____

Date: _____

Principle 2: The Production of Maximum Force

In many sports, athletes are required to use skills that enable them to go "all out" during competition or training. When an athlete applies maximum force, all potential joints that can be used are involved in the movement.

The Vertical Jump

MISSION: Jump as high as possible while varying your jump in the following ways:

   (a) from a standing position
   (b) without using your arms
   (c) without allowing your ankles to plantar flex
   (d) without allowing your trunk to flex at any time

For each jump, record your observations below.

(a) _____

_____

_____

_____

(b) _____

_____

_____

_____

(c) _____

_____

_____

_____

(d) _____

_____

_____

_____

Principle 3: Maximum Velocity: Sequencing of Joint Rotation

The production of maximum velocity requires the use of joints in order from largest to smallest. In performing high-velocity skills, it is usually the larger, slower joints (i.e., those in the leg) that begin the movement while the smaller joints play their role when the preceding joint has reached its peak speed.

Summation of Joint Forces

MISSION: Complete the movements described in the chart below and then record your observations and a rationale for each set of observations.

Movements	Observations	Rationale
Throw a ball... (a) as you normally would, that is, by moving your shoulder to begin the throw (b) with your arm in an outstretched position		
Run as fast as you can... (a) with your arms held firmly at your sides (b) with your arms moving		

Comparison of Joint Movements

MISSION: Repeat Mission 2, but this time select two other skills from a sport or physical activity with which you are familiar. Perform movements to compare the execution of the skill (a) with all the joints that are normally involved in executing that movement, and then (b) without all the joints that are normally involved in executing that movement.

Record your observations in the chart below and provide a rationale for any differences that you observe.

Movements	Observations	Rationale
_____ (a) (b)		
_____ (a) (b)		

12.4 Principles 4 and 5: Linear Motion

According to biomechanical principle 4, the greater the applied impulse, the greater the increase in velocity. Biomechanical principle 5 states that movement usually occurs in the direction opposite that of the applied force.

Name: _____

Date: _____

Important Concepts to Help You Complete This Exercise

- Linear motion is movement in a straight line.
- Momentum refers to the amount of motion developed by an athlete (or object).
- Linear momentum is the amount of momentum developed by an object or body moving in a straight line, a quantity that can be calculated by multiplying the mass of the athlete (or object) by its velocity.
- Impulse refers to the application of force over a period of time that results in a change in momentum.
- Movement usually occurs in the direction opposite that of the applied force.

MISSION: Perform and compare the following three sprint start positions as they relate to the maximal applied force (biomechanical principle 4), the direction of the applied force (biomechanical principle 5), and the resultant force (i.e., the movement outcome or performance). Sketch each position in the second column of the chart, using coloured arrows to indicate the "applied force direction" of the sprinter (you) and the "reaction force direction" of the ground. (Use one colour for the applied force direction and another colour or your choice for the reaction force direction.) Be sure to indicate the angle of each force accurately when drawing it.

In the third column of the chart, describe in point form one or more activity-specific or sport-specific example(s) of the biomechanical principle in action.

Start Position	Sketch	Examples
Standing start Body upright, both feet on the ground, knees slightly bent		
Crouching start Back positioned at a 45 degree angle, knees bent, front foot flat, back foot heel up		
Block start Body bent over, fingers on ground, both heels off ground		

MISSION: Answer the following questions related to biomechanical principles 4 and 5.

1. Identify and explain which of Newton's laws is applied in the performance of each of the sprint starts.

    Standing start

    _____
    _____
    _____

    Crouching start

    _____
    _____
    _____

    Block start

    _____
    _____
    _____
    _____

2. Decide whether your results support biomechanical principle 4: "The greater the applied impulse, the greater the increase in velocity." Explain your answer.

    _____
    _____
    _____
    _____

3. How do starting blocks aid a sprinter? (Hint: Think about balance, gravity, and line of gravity.)

    _____
    _____
    _____

4. List two sports with which you are familiar and in which the direction of force application and/or impulse are important. Identify in which direction the force is being applied to cause the resultant motion. Explain whether your observations support biomechanical principle 5, which states that movement usually occurs in the direction opposite that of the applied force.

    (a) _____
    _____
    _____
    _____

    (b) _____
    _____
    _____
    _____

WORKSHEET

12.5 Principles 6 and 7: Angular Motion

Angular (or rotational) motion is movement around an axis. Our joints serve as axes of rotation for the movement of our limbs. The entire human body can also rotate freely as it moves about one (or more) anatomical axes.

Name: _____

Date: _____

Principle 6: The Production of Angular Motion (Torque)

If an eccentric or "off-centre" force is applied to a body or an object, the force tends to make the body rotate about its axis. This turning effect is known as torque. When a force is applied at some distance from an axis, the turning effect—or torque—results in angular motion.

MISSION: With biomechanical principle 6 in mind, answer questions 1 to 7 below by choosing the correct key term from the ones provided. Terms can be used more than once.

joints   length of the lever arm   vertical   opponent   horizontal

angle at which the force is applied to the lever arm

axis   force   magnitude of the applied force   torque

1. Angular motion is the circular motion that occurs about a(n) _____ of rotation.

2. The application of a _____ acting at some distance from an axis of rotation produces angular motion.

3. The human body is usually described as having three main axes: a _____ axis running through the centre of the body from head to toe (the longitudinal axis); a _____ axis passing from side to side through the centre of the body; and another _____ axis that passes from back to front (the anteroposterior axis).

4. The segments of our bodies have many axes of rotation that permit the movement of our limbs; these axes are known as _____.

5. In some sports such as rugby or football, a(n) _____ imparts an off-centre force in the form of body contact.

6. If the _____ generated at any point of a movement places excessive strain on a tendon, a condition known as tendonitis can result.

7. The three factors that determine the amount of torque generated when a force is applied at some distance from an object's or body's centre of mass are: the _____, the _____, and the _____.

Principle 7: The Conservation of Angular Momentum

Many physical activities and sports require individuals to control the rotation of their bodies while they are airborne and in a state of free fall. When an individual or an object is free in the air, angular momentum is constant. The law of conservation of momentum states that the total angular momentum of a rotating body remains constant if the net torque acting on the rotating body is zero.

MISSION: With biomechanical principle 7 in mind, answer the questions below.

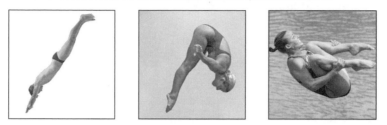

1. In the sport of diving, the basic body positions are layout, pike, and tuck, as shown from left to right above. For each position shown, think about the angular momentum that the diver's body generates. Angular momentum is the product of the diver's rate of rotation (angular velocity) and the extent to which the diver's body resists angular motion (the moment of inertia). The farther a body's distribution of mass is from the axis of rotation, the greater the body's moment of inertia (resistance to angular motion). Taking biomechanical principle 7 into account, determine in which position the diver will rotate most rapidly. Explain your thinking.

Layout: _____

_____

Pike: _____

_____

Tuck: _____

_____

2. In order to achieve the most success once an athlete becomes airborne, when must rotation be initiated? Explain your thinking in terms of biomechanical principle 7.

_____

_____

3. During a dismount from a balance beam, a gymnast attempts to complete as many longitudinal rotations as possible before landing feet first on the mat. (a) What is the best way for the gymnast to initiate the twisting motion? Explain your thinking. (b) How should the gymnast's body be positioned in order to twist most efficiently? Explain your thinking.

(a) _____

(b) _____

4. A common mistake that aerial skiers make when doing difficult tricks is to over-rotate and miss the landing. This mistake can potentially lead to an accident and serious bodily injury. Think about how a coach could explain biomechanical principle 7 to an aerial skier in order to help prevent the skier from being injured. Then answer these questions: (a) How is angular motion generated, and how could it have both positive and negative outcomes in the execution of an aerial trick? (b) How can aerial skiers control their rate of rotation once airborne? (Hint: Consider the potential rotation of a skier's body in all planes.)

(a)_____

(b)_____

WORKSHEET

12.6 Applying the Seven Principles of Biomechanics

Understanding and applying the seven principles of biomechanics can lead to improved motor skills, enhanced athletic performance, and reduced injuries and accidents at work sites.

Name: _____

Date: _____

MISSION: Perform each lab activity with a partner (or in a small group) and answer the accompanying "Biomechanically Speaking ..." reflection question. Then identify which of the seven principles of biomechanics applies to each lab activity, and be sure to use each principle only once. A sample entry is provided below.

Equipment needed: Clothing and footwear appropriate for physical education class, basketballs, measuring tape, pylons, footballs, and floor hockey sticks and balls.

Lab Activity	Biomechanically Speaking...	Biomechanical Principle
Stand with your feet together while your partner gently pushes against your shoulder.	... what can you do to be more stable and resist falling over? Lower my centre of mass—either by bending my knees or spreading my feet apart more.	Principle # 1: STABILITY: The greater the mass, the lower the centre of mass to the base of support, the larger the base of support, and the closer the centre of mass is positioned to the base of support, the more stability increases.
1. Stand behind the foul line and, using only your shoulder, elbow, and wrist joints, try to get a basketball in the basket.		
2. Run as fast as you can for about 20 metres with your arms pressed against your sides.		

3. Using a floor hockey stick and ball, attempt a slapshot using only a 30 cm wind-up.		
4. Throw a perfect spiral with a football.		
5. Perform a modified or standard push-up slowly.		
6. In your stocking feet, spin on one foot, keeping your arms away from your body.		

Chapter 12 Quiz

The two sets of questions below will test your knowledge and broaden your understanding of the material covered in Chapter 12. Complete each set of questions according to your teacher's instructions.

Name: _____

Date: _____

Question Set 1: Principle 1 (Stability) and Principles 2 and 3 (Maximum Effort)

Multiple-Choice Questions

MISSION: Circle the letter beside the answer that you believe to be correct.

1. The branch of mechanics that studies changes in the motion of objects or bodies as a result of the actions of forces acting on them is known as
   (a) statics
   (b) dynamics
   (c) biomechanics
   (d) physics

2. How stable or balanced an individual is while performing a task depends on
   (a) the mass and the centre of mass
   (b) the base of support
   (c) the position of the centre of mass
   (d) all of the above

3. The imaginary middle point around which the mass of an object or a person is balanced is the
   (a) base of support
   (b) centre of mass
   (c) position of the centre of mass
   (d) line of gravity

4. The use of all possible joint movements that contribute to a task's objectives results in
   (a) the production of maximum speed
   (b) the production of maximum effort
   (c) the production of maximum force
   (d) the production of maximum inertia

5. The use of joints in order—from largest to smallest—results in the production of maximum
   (a) speed
   (b) acceleration
   (c) velocity
   (d) all of the above

6. When athletes "give it their all" or "go all out," they are often applying
   (a) biomechanical principle 1
   (b) biomechanical principle 2
   (c) biomechanical principle 3
   (d) both (b) and (c) are correct

Short-Answer Questions

MISSION: Briefly answer the following questions in the space provided:

1. What are the four broad categories into which the seven principles of biomechanics can be grouped?

2. Explain the difference between a static system and a dynamic system.

3. With regard to biomechanical principle 2, what are the consequences if full joint range of motion is restricted at a joint, e.g., due to injury or disease?

Essay Questions

MISSION: On a separate piece of paper, develop a 100-word response to the following questions.

1. How can an understanding of biomechanical principles help movement professionals, athletes, and you yourself to improve your own or someone else's movement proficiency?

2. Use the example of a gymnast on a balance beam to explain what the gymnast can do to improve stability (biomechanical principle 1).

3. Describe how you could apply biomechanical principles 2 and 3 to improve your tennis serve, golf swing, or baseball pitch.

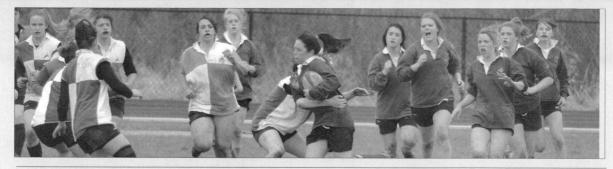

Courtesy of Tanya Winter

Question Set 2: Principles 4 and 5 (Linear Motion) and Principles 6 and 7 (Angular Motion)

Multiple-Choice Questions

MISSION: Circle the letter beside the answer that you believe to be correct.

1. Impulse (the application of a force over a period of time) equals
   (a) mass multiplied by velocity
   (b) mass multiplied by acceleration
   (c) force multiplied by time
   (d) velocity multiplied by acceleration

2. The amount of torque generated depends on the
   (a) magnitude of the applied force
   (b) length of the lever arm (the distance from the point of application of the force and the axis)
   (c) angle at which force is applied to the lever arm
   (d) all of the above

3. Momentum—the quantity of motion contained within an object or body—is equal to
   (a) the object's mass multiplied by its velocity
   (b) the object's mass multiplied by acceleration
   (c) force multiplied by time
   (d) velocity multiplied by acceleration

4. The moment of inertia is defined as
   (a) the distribution of the mass of an object in relation to the axis of rotation
   (b) change in an object's angular velocity
   (c) an object or body's resistance to a change in its rate of angular rotation
   (d) an object's change in direction of movement

5. Angular velocity is
   (a) a quantitative expression
   (b) also called rotational velocity
   (c) the amount of rotation that a spinning object undergoes per unit of time
   (d) all of the above

6. If a diver opens up from a tuck position before entering the pool, the diver's moment of inertia
   (a) increases
   (b) decreases
   (c) neither increases nor decreases
   (d) none of the above

Short-Answer Questions

MISSION: Briefly answer the following questions in the space provided:

1. Which biomechanical principle is closely related to Newton's third law of motion?

2. According to biomechanical principle 6, how is angular or rotational motion produced?

3. When rotations are introduced into a gymnast's routine, what is generated as a result?

Essay Questions

MISSION: On a separate piece of paper, develop a 100-word response to the following questions.

1. Discuss, with examples, the prevalence of biomechanical principles 4, 5, and 6 in everyday life as well as in sports.

2. Mimic a sport skill involving a predominantly rotational motion. Explain how biomechanical principles 6 and 7 apply to the successful execution of that movement.

3. Explain the concept of the conservation of angular momentum, with examples.

WORKSHEET

My Notes on Chapter 12

Use the space below to make notes on the
questions on the facing page, to record any
thoughts and ideas you have on this chapter,
and to store study tips to help you prepare for
tests and exams.

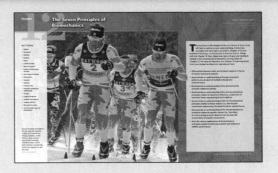

Chapter 12 Review (Student Textbook page 355)

Knowledge

1. Define the terms "static system" and "dynamic system." Give two examples of each type of system.

2. Name and describe the characteristics of two types of static systems. In any static system, what adjective describes the rate of motion of an object or body, whether the object or body is stationary or in motion?

3. Biomechanical principles 2 and 3 pertain to maximizing joint movement and using joints in a certain order to achieve maximum effort. State these two biomechanical principles in your own words.

4. Provide three clear examples from the world of sport in which the sequencing of joint movements is important in achieving maximum effort.

5. In outer space, in theory, a slap shot would propel a puck in a straight line and the puck would continue on that straight-line path forever. What factors prevent a puck from travelling in a straight line forever on Earth?

6. Greater impulse leads to greater velocity. Explain the "impulse-momentum relationship" (i.e., biomechanical principle 4) in your own words and give three examples of this relationship.

7. Define the term "torque" and list three factors that affect the amount of torque generated by the application of an eccentric (off-centre) force to an object.

8. What two variables determine the angular momentum of an individual or object that is rotating freely in the air?

Thinking and Inquiry

9. If a person's base of support is broad and their centre of mass is low and within the base of support, will the person's stability increase or decrease? Refer to biomechanical principle 1 in your answer.

10. Stability is an important feature in most physical movements that occur in sports. However, some sports involve putting yourself in an unstable situation, and then recovering from it. Give three examples of such situations.

11. Do you think it would be advisable to try to apply biomechanical principles 2 and 3 in coaching a four-year-old T-ball player? Explain your answer.

12. How might you modify your hitting or kicking technique to achieve better results in a sport as a result of applying biomechanical principle 4?

13. Using your understanding of bone-muscle anatomy and the production of angular motion according to biomechanical principle 6, analyze how muscle and tendon injury can result from poor technique and/or from the application of excessive force at a joint during the execution of a skill.

Communication

14. Draw a sketch of a four-point stance in football. Label the player's centre of mass and base of support. Write a caption for your drawing.

15. Prepare a presentation explaining the principles of biomechanics with sport-specific examples.

16. Scan the sports section of a newspaper or magazine or watch a sports event on TV or online, looking for examples of biomechanical principle 5 in action. Prepare a brief summary of your observations.

17. Figure skaters or divers can control their rate of rotation by moving their arms closer to or farther from their body. Write a paragraph or draw a labelled sketch of how this action reflects an application of biomechanical principle 7.

Application

18. Falling is a leading cause of early death among seniors. What advice based on biomechanical principle 1 could you offer to senior family members who might be a little "wobbly" on their feet?

19. In a group of three, take turns demonstrating a tennis stroke, a soccer kick, and an underhand softball pitch. Analyze the movements orally or in writing with reference to biomechanical principles 2 and 3.

20. Tennis coaches working with young children, who do not normally exert a lot of hitting power, often use softer balls. In terms of the Impulse-momentum relationship, what does this achieve, and why is it likely to help?

21. Choose a joint in the human body (e.g., shoulder, ankle, or knee) and simulate a sport movement that involves that joint primarily. While demonstrating the movement, describe the factors that affect the amount of torque generated through the joint's full range of motion.

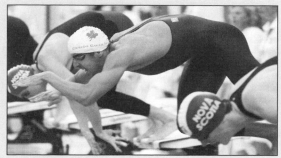

Team Ontario swimmer Hassaan Abdel Khalik pushes off the start line in the men's 50-metre freestyle at the Canada Games in Charlottetown in 2009, demonstrating biomechanical principle 5. (CP Photo/Andrew Vaughan)

Analyzing the Efficiency of Human Movement

KEY TERMS

- Functional movement
- Energy leaks
- Qualitative analysis
- Quantitative analysis
- Motion-capture system

Canada's Todd Nicholson celebrates with team members after winning the gold medal at the end of the Sledge Ice Hockey final between Canada and Norway at the 2006 Winter Paralympic games in Turin, Italy.

CP Photo Archive/AP/Alberto Ramella

> "Science requires an engagement with the world, a live encounter between the knower and the known."
>
> —Parker J. Palmer, author and educator

The exercises in this chapter of the *Lab Manual & Study Guide* will help to reinforce your understanding of some key concepts and main topics covered in Chapter 13 of your textbook *Kinesiology: An Introduction to Exercise Science*. Along with the Chapter 13 Quiz, these exercises will give you feedback related to the achievement of selected Learning Goals for Chapter 13. For ease of reference, the Chapter 13 Learning Goals from your student textbook are reproduced here:

- differentiate between a qualitative and quantitative biomechanical analysis

- demonstrate an understanding of how biomechanists and other movement professionals conduct qualitative analyses, quantitative analyses, or a combination of both types of analysis to assess human movement

- demonstrate an understanding of how qualitative and quantitative analysis can be used to counteract disruptions in the efficiency of human movement

- describe the advantages and limitations of qualitative biomechanical analysis

- describe the advantages and limitations of quantitative biomechanical analysis

- demonstrate an understanding of the various purposes and applications of biomechanical movement analyses, e.g., to enhance elite athletic performance

- use the appropriate laws of physics and/or biomechanical principles to analyze the efficiency of a movement pattern during physical activity

WORKSHEET

13.1 Qualitative Analysis

Coaches use qualitative analysis to break down a skill in order to find ways to improve proficiency in the execution of that skill.

MISSION: Complete the table using the biomechanical concepts and principles you have learned to date.

Name: _____

Date: _____

(A) A Slapshot in Hockey

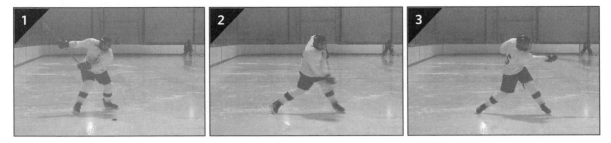

Record and Explain: Examine the hockey slapshot sequence shown in the photographs above. Now begin to analyze the sequence using some of the biomechanical terminology you have learned.

Divide up into groups of 3-5 students. Take turns replicating the skill movement as best you can, helping others with the execution of the skill if they need it.

In the table below, using biomechanical terms, write in your observations about the mechanics of the skill through its key phases. Suggest ways that execution of a slapshot or similar skill (a tennis forehand, for example) can be improved by applying a basic understanding of biomechanical concepts and principles.

Phase of Movement	Qualitative Observations Using Biomechanical Concepts and Principles
1. Preliminary movements	
2. Execution	
3. Follow-through	

QUALITATIVE ANALYSIS
(B) A Soccer Kick

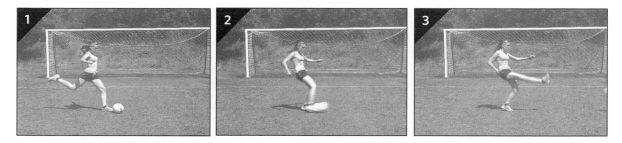

Record and Explain: Examine the soccer kick sequence shown in the photographs above. Now begin to analyze the sequence using some of the biomechanical terminology you have learned.

Divide up into groups of 3-5 students. Take turns replicating the skill movement as best you can, helping others with the execution of the skill if they need it.

In the table below, using biomechanical terms, write your observations about the mechanics of the skill through its key phases. Suggest ways that execution of a soccer kick or a similar skill (a punt in football, for example), can be improved by applying a basic understanding of biomechanical concepts and principles.

Phase of Movement	Qualitative Observations Using Biomechanical Concepts and Principles
1. Preliminary movements	
2. Execution	
3. Follow-through	

QUALITATIVE ANALYSIS
(C) A Golf Stroke

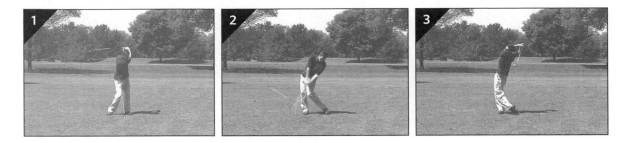

Record and Explain: Examine the golf stroke sequence shown in the photographs above. Now begin to analyze the sequence using some of the biomechanical terminology you have learned.

Divide up into groups of 3-5 students. Take turns replicating the skill movement as best you can, helping others with the execution of the skill if they need it.

In the table below, using biomechanical terms, write in some observations about the mechanics of the stroke through its key phases. Suggest ways that execution of a golf stroke or a similar skill (a backhand in tennis, for example), can be improved by applying a basic understanding of biomechanical concepts and principles.

Phase of Movement	Qualitative Observations Using Biomechanical Concepts and Principles
1. Preliminary movements	
2. Execution	
3. Follow-through	

QUALITATIVE ANALYSIS
(D) A Tennis Serve

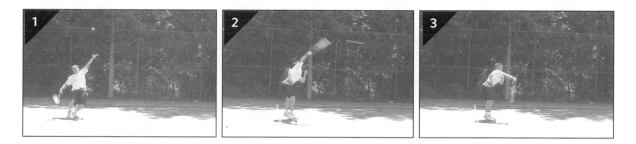

Record and Explain: Examine the tennis serve sequence shown in the photographs above. Now begin to analyze the sequence using some of the biomechanical terminology you have learned.

Divide up into groups of 3-5 students. Take turns replicating the skill movement as best you can, helping others with the execution of the skill if they need it.

In the table below, using biomechanical terms, write in some observations about the mechanics of the serve through its key phases. Suggest ways that execution of a tennis serve or a similar skill (a volleyball smash, for example), can be improved by applying a basic understanding of biomechanical concepts and principles.

Phase of Movement	Qualitative Observations Using Biomechanical Concepts and Principles
1. Preliminary movements	
2. Execution	
3. Follow-through	

13.2 Determining the Position of the Centre of Mass

The centre of mass plays an important part in biomechanical analysis, but this position can be difficult to locate precisely in the human body. The "segmentation method" is one way to estimate the location of the centre of mass.

Name: _____

Date: _____

Can a force such as gravity be considered to act through a single point in the body? The answer is "yes" and this point is called the "centre of mass."

If the object is of uniform density and shape, then this point will be in the geometric centre of the object. However, a different method must be used to compute the position of the centre of mass of the human body (which is not uniform in density or shape).

To find the position of the centre of mass of the human body, it is necessary first to determine the position of the centre of mass of each body segment. This method is referred to as the segmentation method.

Note that the position of the centre of mass of a human body need not fall within the boundaries of the body. Rather, the position is dependent upon the orientation of the arms and legs.

Segment	Centre of Mass Position
Head	46% (from the top)
Trunk	38% (from the neck)
Upper Arm	51% (from the shoulder)
Forearm	39% (from the elbow)
Hand	82% (from the wrist)
Thigh	37% (from the hip)
Calf (shank)	37% (from the knee)
Foot	45% (from the heel)

These percentages were provided by Professor David Sanderson at the University of British Columbia. They can be used to estimate the segmental centres of mass. Other biomechanists may use slightly different percentages, but they will arrive at similar results.

MISSION: Compute the position of the centre of mass of the diver in the photo at the top of page 213. To do this, you must first determine the position of the centre of mass of each body segment (using x- and y-coordinates). Follow these steps.

- **STEP 1:** Note that a straight line has been placed over each of the body segments: foot, shank (lower leg), thigh, trunk, head, and left and right upper arm, forearm, and hand. These lines represent a stick figure of the diver. The length of each line segment is given in column A of the table (in centimetres). We can use these lines plus some other measures to determine the position of the whole body centre of mass.

- **STEP 2:** Now, each body segment itself is not of uniform density and shape, so a percentage must be applied to each measurement of length in order to estimate the centre of mass for that segment. These percentages are entered in column B (transferred from the table on this page). Multiply the length of the line by this percentage in order to locate the point of the centre of mass for each body segment. Enter this number in column C for each segment and mark this location with a dot on each line on the photo. Plot this point starting from the correct end of the line (see table on this page).

- **STEP 3:** Once you have pinpointed all the segmental centres of mass, using the lower left corner of the photo as the origin, measure the x- and y-coordinates for each of the points. For each centre of mass, enter these x- and y-coordinates in column D and column E respectively.

- **STEP 4:** Each body segment carries a different importance in relation to the position of the whole-body centre of mass. Again, we must use a "weighting factor" that approximates the significance of each body part on the overall centre of mass. This factor is provided for you in column F. Multiply the value of each x and y coordinate by this factor and enter the values in columns G and H respectively.

- **STEP 5:** Add up the values in column G and enter this in the bottom row. Do the same for column H. Mark this point (the intersection of the x- and y-coordinates) on the photo using an "X". This "X" represents an estimate of the position of the centre of mass for the diver using the segmentation method.

Re-Visiting the Steps

First you need to calculate the position of the centre of mass for each body segment (enter this number in column C in the table below).

Mark a dot on each line to indicate the position of the centre of mass for each body segment. (Be sure to measure from the correct end of the line.)

Find the x- and y-coordinates for each of these points and enter them in columns D and E. Then calculate the adjusted x- and y-coordinates (columns G and H).

Add up the adjusted x- and y-coordinates and you will have the final coordinates for the whole-body centre of mass. (Answers may differ slightly depending on the exact numbers for x- and y-coordinates.)

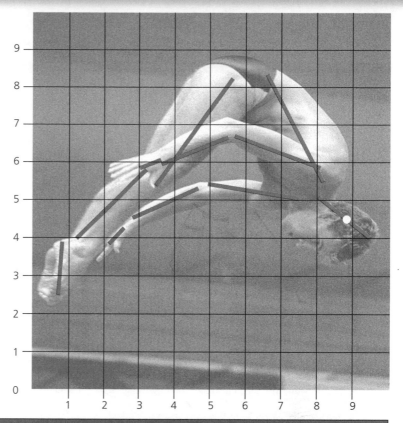

Body Segment	A Length of the Body Segment (provided in cm)	B "Multiplier" To find the Centre of Mass for each Segment	C Distance to Segment's Centre of Mass (in cm) (A x B)	D The x-Coordinate of Centre of Mass of the Segment	E The y-Coordinate of Centre of Mass of the Segment	F "Weighting" Factor for that Body Segment	G Adjusted x-Coordinate (F x D)	H Adjusted y-Coordinate (F x E)
Head	1.7	.46	.782	8.9	4.6	.07	.623	.322
Trunk	3.2	.38				.51		
Right upper arm	2.4	.51				.03		
Right forearm	1.9	.39				.02		
Right hand	.6	.82				.01		
Left upper arm	2.4	.51				.03		
Left forearm	1.9	.39				.02		
Left hand	.6	.82				.01		
Thigh	3.5	.37				.20		
Calf (shank)	2.6	.37				.08		
Foot	1.4	.45				.02		
TOTALS x- and y-coordinates for the diver's centre of mass								

13.3 Measuring Human Motion

Plotting the x- and y-coordinates of joints reveals motion characteristics that can be used in the analysis of human movement.

MISSION: Plot the x- and y-coordinate for the hip, knee, and ankle of the right leg.

Name: _____

Date: _____

To quantify human movement for analysis, the first step is to convert visual images into numeric values. This process is called "digitizing," which simply refers to a method of obtaining an x- and y-coordinate for each joint of interest.

On the adjacent page there are ten sequential photographs of a player kicking a soccer ball. The coordinates for each joint movement are shown.

These values can be used to create a stick figure plot of the kicking movement. Representations like this can then be used by quantitative biomechanists to gain valuable information about the nature of movement at joints (angular velocity, angular acceleration, etc.).

For this exercise, we will simply plot the kicking data.

Use the bottom left corner of the graph below as your graph origin and plot the x- and y-coordinates given for each photograph. Two sample entries are included (photographs 1 and 10 are plotted). Label each stick figure with the photo number.

Note the path of each marker. The foot goes through a much larger movement than the knee and hip. In fact, the hip moves only a small amount and mostly in the forward direction. In general, most physical movement involves large motion at the end of body segments, while the joints closer to the body remain relatively stable.

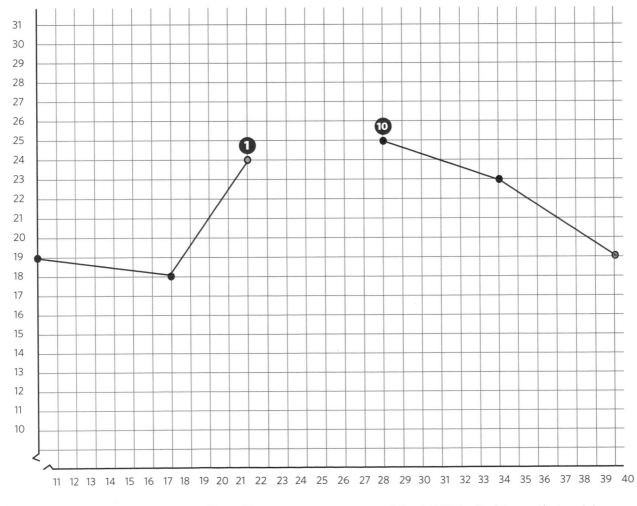

1

Hip
Ankle
Knee

Coordinates in millimetres

	x Axis	y Axis
Hip	21	24
Knee	17	18
Ankle	10	19

2

	x Axis	y Axis
Hip	23	24
Knee	19	16
Ankle	13	21

3

	x Axis	y Axis
Hip	24	23
Knee	23	17
Ankle	16	21

4

	x Axis	y Axis
Hip	26	23
Knee	27	16
Ankle	19	19

5

	x Axis	y Axis
Hip	28	23
Knee	31	16
Ankle	24	15

6

Coordinates in millimetres

	x Axis	y Axis
Hip	25	23
Knee	30	18
Ankle	28	11

7

	x Axis	y Axis
Hip	25	23
Knee	32	17
Ankle	34	10

8

	x Axis	y Axis
Hip	27	23
Knee	33	19
Ankle	38	13

9

	x Axis	y Axis
Hip	27	24
Knee	34	21
Ankle	40	16

10

	x Axis	y Axis
Hip	28	25
Knee	34	23
Ankle	40	19

Photos courtesy of David Sanderson, UBC.

WORKSHEET

Chapter 13 Quiz

The two sets of questions below will test your knowledge and broaden your understanding of the material covered in Chapter 13. Complete each set of questions according to your teacher's instructions.

Name: _____

Date: _____

Question Set 1: Qualitative and Quantitative Biomechanical Analysis

Multiple-Choice Questions

MISSION: Circle the letter beside the answer that you believe to be correct.

1. Qualitative biomechanical analysis typically involves
   (a) data collection
   (b) mathematical analysis
   (c) near-laboratory conditions
   (d) descriptive analysis of movement

2. Which of the following does not apply to qualitative biomechanical analysis?
   (a) little or no equipment is required
   (b) generally does not require data collection and mathematical analysis
   (c) findings can be regarded as evidence-based, authoritative, and unbiased
   (d) allows coaches to interact immediately with participants to help improve their technique

3. Which of the following does not apply to quantitative biomechanical analysis?
   (a) hard data can be collected and analyzed using rigorous mathematical techniques
   (b) results can be verified by other analysts
   (c) findings can be regarded as evidence-based, authoritative, and unbiased
   (d) little or no equipment is required

4. Biomechanists have analyzed Usain Bolt's remarkable feat in the 100-metre sprint using quantitative means. They were able to determine
   (a) the amount of drag (air resistance) he encountered as he ran
   (b) how much energy he used to finish the race
   (c) the maximum power he generated as he ran
   (d) all of the above

5. Measuring joint angles during a soccer kick using motion-capture videorecording and calculating angular velocity is an example of:
   (a) qualitative analysis
   (b) quantitative analysis
   (c) both quantitative and qualitative analysis
   (d) neither quantitative nor qualitative analysis

Short-Answer Questions

MISSION: Briefly answer the following questions in the space provided:

1. Define the term "efficiency of movement" and give an example of an efficient movement.

2. Explain what is meant by the term "functional movement."

3. What is the essential difference between qualitative and quantitative biomechanical analysis?

Essay Questions

MISSION: On a separate piece of paper, develop a 100-word response to the following questions.

1. Think of a sport skill that you are familiar with (e.g., a chest pass in basketball). Explain what might constitute (a) a qualitative analysis and (b) a quantitative analysis of that skill.

2. Explain how "Own the Podium" relies heavily on quantitative analysis to achieve its goals.

3. Which type of analysis (qualitative or quantitative) would you feel more comfortable using to improve your performance in a physical activity or sport? Explain your answer.

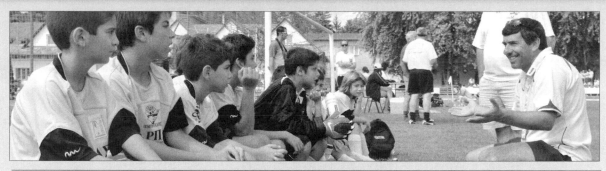

Muzsy/Shutterstock

Question Set 2: Applying Biomechanical Concepts and Principles in Analyzing Human Movement

Multiple-Choice Questions

MISSION: Circle the letter beside the answer that you believe to be correct.

1. Which biomechanical principle would feature prominently in the case of lifting a bag of groceries off the floor?
   (a) stability (#1)
   (b) the impulse-momentum relationship (#4)
   (c) torque (#6)
   (d) conservation of angular momentum (#7)

2. Which biomechanical principle would feature prominently in the case of a child beginning to walk?
   (a) stability (#1)
   (b) the impulse-momentum relationship (#4)
   (c) torque (#6)
   (d) conservation of angular momentum (#7)

3. Which biomechanical principle would feature prominently in the case of a trampolinist doing a spin in the air?
   (a) stability (# 1)
   (b) the impulse-momentum relationship (#4)
   (c) torque (#6)
   (d) conservation of angular momentum (#7)

4. Which biomechanical principle would feature prominently in the case of screwing in a lightbulb?
   (a) stability (#1)
   (b) the impulse-momentum relationship (#4)
   (c) torque (#6)
   (d) conservation of angular momentum (#7)

5. Which biomechanical principle would feature prominently in the case of pitching a ball?
   (a) stability (#1)
   (b) the impulse-momentum relationship (#4)
   (c) torque (#6)
   (d) conservation momentum (#7)

Short-Answer Questions

MISSION: Briefly answer the following questions in the space provided:

1. List three biomechanical concepts and/or principles demonstrated by a toddler who is learning to walk.

2. State the most noticeable biomechanical difference between a proficient soccer player and a beginner.

3. How can a shooter increase the amount of momentum and the velocity imparted to a puck when taking a wrist shot in floor hockey?

Essay Questions

MISSION: On a separate piece of paper, develop a 100-word response to the following questions.

1. Summarize the biomechanical concepts and principles involved when a player kicks a soccer ball.

2. Explain the importance of ground reaction force and biomechanical principle 5 in floor hockey and in a sport of your choice.

3. Describe the general benefits of computerized motion analysis for coaches, teachers, students, and athletes at all levels.

My Notes on Chapter 13

Use the space below to make notes on the questions on the facing page, to record any thoughts and ideas you have on this chapter, and to store study tips to help you prepare for tests and exams.

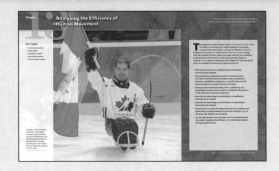

Chapter 13 Review (Student Textbook page 371)

Knowledge

1. A knowledge of biomechanics can improve the efficiency and proficiency with which one executes a skill. Distinguish between the terms "efficiency" and "proficiency."

2. Biomechanists often use the term "disrupted movement patterns." What does this term mean? How does this concept relate to occupational therapy, rehabilitation work with seniors, or work with persons with disabilities?

3. The biomechanics of walking is fairly complex. Describe some of the variables that biomechanists observe when performing a gait analysis.

4. What are the primary differences, biomechanically speaking, between a child learning to walk, a mature adult walker, and a senior citizen who may be having trouble "getting around"?

5. From a biomechanical perspective, explain how a floor hockey player could generate more power from a wrist shot.

6. What is meant by "computerized motion analysis" and what are some of its applications? What kinds of measurements does computerized motion analysis allow that otherwise would be difficult to achieve by sensory observational analysis?

Thinking and Inquiry

7. Most professional biomechanists have a background in physics, mathematics, or a related field, but biomechanists use both qualitative and quantitative methods in analyzing human movement patterns. Compare and contrast qualitative and quantitative methods of analyzing functional movement.

8. Some biomechanical problems lend themselves to a quantitative approach, while others lend themselves to a qualitative approach. Give an example of situations in which each approach is used and for which the alternative method of analysis might be completely unsuitable.

9. What factors play a role in a successful penalty kick in soccer? Describe the biomechanics involved in making this kind of kick in soccer, from start to finish. Explain what a player would need to do to "bend it like Beckham."

10. Do you think that computerized video analysis would benefit elite athletes more than novice athletes? Why or why not?

11. Many computerized motion analysis systems are portable, allowing instant feedback in live-action situations. What are the advantages of this type of "on-the-field" analysis?

Communication

12. With the help of a coach or a physical education teacher, conduct a qualitative analysis of a selected movement pattern demonstrated by a friend or a classmate. Prepare a brief written record of your analysis using biomechanical terms, concepts, and principles.

13. In a graphic organizer of your choice, show the advantages and disadvantages of qualitative analysis versus quantitative analysis in biomechanics.

14. Create a series of simple drawings showing the events involved in a wrist shot in floor hockey. Highlight areas where slight modifications to one's technique could impart greater velocity to the puck, greater stability during execution, and greater accuracy.

Application

15. Applying the biomechanical concepts and principles you learned in this unit, suggest ways to improve your proficiency in the performance of an everyday physical activity such as bending to pick up a heavy item, riding a bicycle, or climbing a ladder.

16. Repeat a series of striking movements (for example, a tennis serve), but vary one component of your stroke each time, for example, how you hold your racquet, how much impulse you deliver, how far above your head you hit the ball, and so on. Before you strike the object, apply your knowledge of biomechanics to predict what the outcome will be as a result of modifying your stroke. Repeat each variation several times. Compare the results against your predictions.

17. Ask a friend or classmate to use a video camera to record your performance of a sport skill in which you are somewhat proficient. Using the slow motion and freeze-frame features, analyze your movement applying the seven biomechanical principles and knowledge of anatomy. Evaluate whether the video analysis helped improve your level of proficiency.

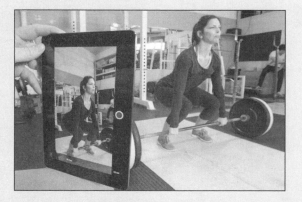

Computerized motion analysis is used to capture Canadian snowboarder Caroline Calvé's movements during her training in Montréal for the Sochi Winter Olympics in 2014. (CP Photo/Paul Chiasson)

UNIT 3: HUMAN PERFORMANCE AND BIOMECHANICS

Career Choices

Investigate a career in one of the fields mentioned in this unit. Ideally, you should interview someone working within the field for this assignment. You can ask him or her the following questions and a lot more as well.

Name: _____

Date: _____

MISSION: Answer the series of questions below in relation to the career you have selected. If you interviewed a person for this career information, use quotation marks to distinguish what they said from your own comments on the career. Give the person's name and job title.

1 Career and description

_____

_____

_____

_____

_____

2 List at least two post-secondary institutions in Ontario and/or Canada that offer programs for this career.

_____

_____

_____

_____

3 Choose one of the above institutions and determine the required courses in the first year of study for this program.

_____

_____

_____

_____

4 How many years of post-secondary education are required before beginning this career? Is an internship or apprenticeship required?

_____

_____

_____

_____

5 What is the demand for individuals qualified for this occupation? If possible, provide some employment data to support your answer.

_____

_____

_____

_____

6 What is the average starting salary for this career? What is the top salary? On what do salary increases depend in this career?

_____

_____

_____

_____

7 List occupational settings where a person with these qualifications could work.

_____

_____

_____

_____

Nutrition for Human Performance

The quality and timing of nutritional intake—including fluid intake—is of critical importance in maximizing your performance on and off the playing field.

Sebastian Duda/Shutterstock

The exercises in this chapter of the *Lab Manual & Study Guide* will help to reinforce your understanding of some key concepts and main topics covered in Chapter 14 of your textbook *Kinesiology: An Introduction to Exercise Science*. Along with the Chapter 14 Quiz, these exercises will give you feedback related to the achievement of selected Learning Goals for Chapter 14. For ease of reference, the Chapter 14 Learning Goals from your student textbook are reproduced here:

- describe the relationship between nutrition and human performance and the importance of nutritional awareness for athletes and those who are physically active

- identify dietary sources of macronutrients (proteins, carbohydrates, fats, water) and micronutrients (vitamins and minerals) and explain their functions in the body

- explain the features and benefits of Canada's Food Guide along with Health Canada's Dietary Reference Intakes and regulation of food labelling

- explain how the "energy equation" helps to maintain a healthy body weight by balancing energy intake and energy expenditure

- estimate one's daily caloric need based on calculating resting metabolic rate

- analyze the problem of obesity and inactivity in Canada and explain how Body Mass Index (BMI) is used to assess whether a person is obese, overweight, or underweight

- understand the importance of a combined approach to altering body weight or composition through appropriate caloric intake and physical activity

- describe the components of the female athlete triad (low energy availability, menstrual irregularities, bone disease)

- modify dietary intake to match performance requirements

- monitor fluid replacement before, during, and after exercise to avoid dehydration, muscle cramps, heat stroke, heat exhaustion, and hyponatremia

WORKSHEET

14.1 Creating a Nutrition Facts Label for a Smoothie

Making healthy food choices and learning how to achieve the right nutritional balance is key to maintaining a healthy body weight, ensuring sufficient energy for daily activities, and furthering your goal of optimal performance.

Name: _____

Date: _____

MISSION: Fill in the following table and then complete the templates on the next page.

Step 1: In a small group (2–5 students), choose from the ingredients listed in the table below to make a blended smoothie. (You may use different food items upon the approval of your teacher.) Complete the table by filling in the required information for each of the ingredients listed.

Step 2: On the following page, complete the food label by providing the nutritional information related to your smoothie.

Step 3: Create a product name as well as a brief promotional description that focusses on the nutritional value that your smoothie provides.

Tip: Use the following website to acquire your nutritional food values:

http://www.eatwise.ca (Dietitians of Canada)

Ingredient	Approx. Grams Used	Carbo-hydrate per Gram	Fat per Gram	Protein per gram	Total Energy	Choles-terol	Sodium	Vitamin A	Vitamin C	Calcium	Iron	Fibre
Ice cream												
Yoghurt												
Banana												
Apple												
Chocolate syrup												
Pineapple juice												
Kiwi												
Strawberry												
Cantaloupe												
Peach												
Watermelon												
Totals												

Nutrition Facts

Per _____ mL (_____ g)

Amount   % Daily Value

Calories _____

Fat _____ g   _____ %

   Saturated _____ g
   + Trans _____ g   _____ %

Cholesterol _____ mg

Sodium _____ mg   _____ %

Carbohydrate _____ g   _____ %

   Fibre _____ g   _____ %

   Sugars _____ g

Protein _____ g

Vitamin A _____ %   Vitamin C _____ %

Calcium _____ %   Iron _____ %

Descriptive Label for Your Smoothie

_____

_____

_____

_____

_____

14.2 Estimating RMR and Daily Caloric Need

By determining your resting metabolic rate (RMR), it is possible to determine the daily caloric need required to sustain your current healthy body weight.

Name: _____

Date: _____

MISSION: Follow steps 1 and 2 to complete the table.

Step 1:
Use the Harris-Benedict equation (provided below) to calculate your own resting metabolic rate (RMR). Insert the required information (height, weight, and age) in the appropriate table below.

Step 2:
Estimate your daily caloric need as follows: multiply RMR by 1.4 if you are sedentary; multiply RMR by 1.6 if you are moderately active; multiply RMR by 1.8 if you engage in hard exercise or vigorous sports.

RMR = constant + (___× ht. in cm) + (___× wt. in kg) – (___× age)

Resting Metabolic Rate for Males					
Constant					66.5
Height	5	×		cm	+
Weight	13.7	×		kg	+
				Subtotal	
Age	6.8	×		yrs	–
				RESTING METABOLIC RATE =	

Resting Metabolic Rate for Females					
Constant					66.5
Height	1.9	×		cm	+
Weight	9.5	×		kg	+
				Subtotal	
Age	4.7	×		yrs	–
				RESTING METABOLIC RATE =	

RMR		Activity Factor	Daily Caloric Need
	×		kcal/day

WORKSHEET

14.3 Tracking Daily Caloric Intake

Eating wisely is only one step in the process of achieving optimal performance. It is necessary to match your daily energy intake with your daily energy needs.

Name: _____

Date: _____

MISSION: Do steps 1-3 to check your energy balance.

Step 1: In the chart provided on the next two pages, record your food intake for a two-day period. In the shaded areas, indicate the total calories (energy intake) and then divide by 2 to compute your average daily caloric intake. In the first row below, insert your average daily caloric intake.

Step 2: In the second row in the table below, insert your estimated daily caloric need (previously calculated in Exercise 14.2).

Step 3: To estimate your energy surplus or shortfall based on these values, subtract your estimated daily caloric need from your average daily caloric intake.

Note: If the difference between the two values is great, speculate as to why there is a large difference—perhaps you are more active than you realized (or perhaps you need to be more active).

Your food values for Step 1 can be obtained from: http://www.eatwise.ca (Dietitians of Canada).

Average daily caloric intake	
Estimated daily caloric need	
Energy surplus or shortfall =	

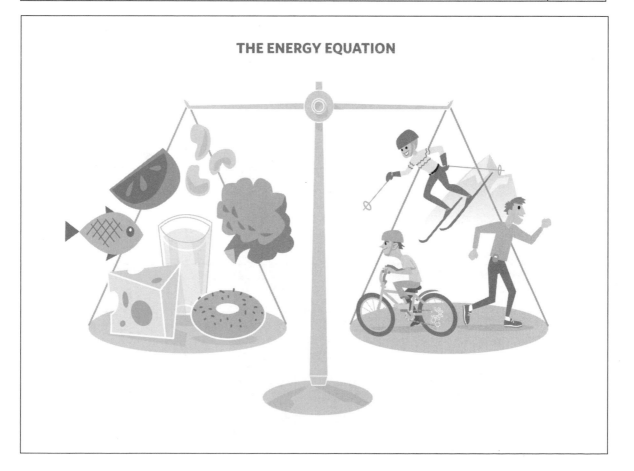

THE ENERGY EQUATION

Food	Approx. Grams Used	Carbo-hydrate per Gram	Fat per Gram	Protein per Gram	Total Energy	Vitamins A	C	Calcium	Iron
Day 1 **Food Intake**									
Day 1 Totals									

Food	Approx. Grams Used	Carbo- hydrate per Gram	Fat per Gram	Protein per Gram	Total Energy	Vitamins A	C	Calcium	Iron
Day 2 Food Intake									
Day 2 Totals									
Two-Day Totals									
Average Daily Caloric Intake									

14.4 It's Not All About Calories: Planning a Balanced Diet

Variety in your diet is essential to help ensure optimal physical and mental performance at every level. But how can you achieve the appropriate variety? You can use the Coaching Association of Canada's "Food Group" method.

Name: _____

Date: _____

A Balanced Diet for Optimal Performance

Variety and balance are important when it comes to eating for optimal performance. You need to take in the full range of nutrients your body needs. Calories alone are not enough to sustain you over the long run.

The Coaching Association of Canada recommends considering the "Food Group" method for meal planning to ensure variety.

This Food Group Method can help ensure you get all the nutrients you need in your diet.

The Food Groups

Here are the food groups and the number of servings from each group that the Coaching Association of Canada recommends you consume each day:

- **Grain Products**
  2-6 servings
- **Vegetables and fruit**
  2-6 servings
- **Milk and alternatives**
  1/2-1 serving
- **Meat and alternatives**
  1/2-1 serving
- **Oils and fat**
  3 servings
- **Fluids**
  In sufficient quantities to stay hydrated

MISSION: Create a healthy meal plan for a day that will ensure that there is variety in your diet and also provide the appropriate number of calories for your level of physical activity.

STEPS:

1. The adjacent table shows menu selections for a day's meals. It also shows the food group for each item.

2. Using the meal planner on the following page, indicate first whether you think of yourself as a Level 1 athlete (a beginner), a Level 2 athlete (average), or a Level 3 athlete (advanced). This will affect your overall calorie target range.

3. Use the first column to select your breakfast, lunch, and dinner choices (as well as snacks) for a day. You can vary the quantities and the items. Add other items too, if you like. But make it tasty. The first item is written in for you (but change it, if you wish.)

4. Once you have made your food selections, add up the number of servings from each food group to see if you are achieving variety in your diet and are in the recommended range for each of the food groups.

5. In the final column, add calorie counts to see if you fall into the desired calorie range for your level of activity. You can find calorie counts at: www.eatwise.ca

Menu Selections: The food group designations will help you add variety to your diet.	
Meal/Snacks	**Food Group**
Breakfast	
Small glass of juice	Vegetables and fruit
Whole wheat pancake	Grain products
Blueberries	Vegetables and fruit
Scrambled egg	Meat and alternatives
Small glass of milk	Milk and alternatives
Margarine	Oils and fats
Snacks	
Low-fat muffin	Grain products
Apple or banana	Vegetables and fruit
Lunch	
Pita bread	Grain products
Mayonnaise	Oils and fats
Small portion of tuna	Meat and alternatives
Raw vegetables	Vegetables and fruit
Small glass of milk	Milk and alternatives
Fruit smoothie	Vegetables and fruit
Snacks	
Multi-grain bread	Grain products
Milk	Milk and alternatives
Dinner	
Small portion of beef	Meat and alternatives
Broccoli stir-fry	Vegetables and fruit
Brown rice	Grain products
Mushrooms/celery	Vegetables and fruit
Margarine	Oils and fats
Peaches	Vegetables and fruit
Yogurt topping	Milk and alternatives
Snacks	
Oatmeal cookie	Grain products
Milk-based hot chocolate	Milk & alternatives

My Menu Selections Using the "Food Group" Method						My Athletic Level: ____
	Food Group and Number of Servings					**Approx. Number of Calories**
	Grain Products	**Vegetables and Fruit**	**Milk and Alternatives**	**Meat and Alternatives**	**Oils and Fats**	
BREAKFAST						
Orange juice		1				50
Wholewheat pancake	2					100
Egg			1			100
Snack						
Subtotals (Morning)						
LUNCH						
Snack						
Subtotals (Afternoon)						
DINNER						
Snack						
Subtotals (Evening)						
DAILY TOTALS						

WORKSHEET

Chapter 14 Quiz

The two sets of questions below will test your knowledge and broaden your understanding of the material covered in Chapter 14. Complete each set of questions according to your teacher's instructions.

Name: _____

Date: _____

Question Set 1: Nutrition Basics—Nutrients, Energy Balance, and Body Weight

Multiple-Choice Questions

MISSION: Circle the letter beside the answer that you believe to be correct.

1. Which of the following are macronutrients?
   (a) calcium and iron
   (b) vitamins and minerals
   (c) carbohydrates, proteins, fats, and water
   (d) carbohydrates, proteins, and fats

2. Which of the following statements are true?
   (a) micronutrients include vitamins and minerals.
   (b) micronutrients assist in energy metabolism.
   (c) micronutrients help in tissue synthesis.
   (d) all of the above

3. Health Canada's recommendations as to how much of each nutrient we need each day to stay healthy
   (a) are known as Dietary Reference Intakes
   (b) are known as Nutrition Facts Tables
   (c) are known as the % Daily Value
   (d) are known as Nutrient Content Claims

4. Which of the following vitamins are fat-soluble?
   (a) C, D, and E
   (b) A, B, C, and K
   (c) B and C
   (d) A, D, E, and K

5. Three factors that contribute to daily caloric need are
   (a) basal metabolic rate
   (b) calories needed to fuel activity
   (c) the thermic effect of food
   (d) all of the above

6. The Harris-Benedict equation can help estimate
   (a) the rate at which your cardiovascular system uses energy
   (b) the rate at which all your muscles, taken together, use energy on a daily basis
   (c) the amount of calories you need to consume each day
   (d) a rate of energy consumption that only applies to those who work out

Short-Answer Questions

MISSION: Briefly answer the following questions in the space provided:

1. What happens when we consume carbohydrates in excess amounts?

2. What is the difference between unsaturated fats and saturated fats?

3. What percentages of our daily caloric intake should come from carbohydrates, fats, and proteins?

Essay Questions

MISSION: On a separate piece of paper, develop a 100-word response to the following questions.

1. Explain the principle underlying eating well in order to maintain a healthy body weight in the context of the "energy equation."

2. Describe two common ways to establish a baseline for a weight-control program using diet and exercise.

3. Why should we limit consumption of trans fats?

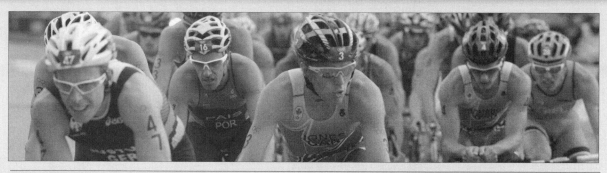

CP Photo/HO, COC—Jason Ransom

Question Set 2: Nutrition and Hydration for Optimal Performance

Multiple-Choice Questions

MISSION: Circle the letter beside the answer that you believe to be correct.

1. The best way to lose body weight is to
   (a) follow a strict diet
   (b) increase physical activity, do some resistance training, and adjust caloric intake
   (c) limit consumption of carbohydrates
   (d) avoid foods that contain fats

2. An athlete's diet should be
   (a) high in protein and high in fat
   (b) low in carbohydrate, low in fat, and varied
   (c) high in protein and electrolytes
   (d) high in carbohydrate, low in fat, and varied

3. A proposed internal control mechanism that tightly maintains body weight and body fat is known as
   (a) set-point theory
   (b) body composition theory
   (c) optimal nutritional intake theory
   (d) total energy expenditure theory

4. The ratio of a person's weight to the square of his or her height is known as
   (a) Glycemic Index
   (b) Body Fat Index
   (c) Body Composition Index
   (d) Body Mass Index

5. Active individuals and athletes need to ensure
   (a) replacement of fluids throughout the day
   (b) all food group servings throughout the day
   (c) balanced meals and snacks throughout the day
   (d) all of the above

6. Roughly what percentage of fluid lost during exercise or training should active individuals and athletes try to consume?
   (a) 75 percent
   (b) 100 percent
   (c) 150 percent
   (d) 200 percent

Short-Answer Questions

MISSION: Briefly answer the following questions in the space provided:

1. What are the three components of the female athlete triad?

2. Why is the timing of nutrient intake by athletes very important?

3. What two main neurological reflexes facilitate the cooling process when our bodies produce heat through exercise?

Essay Questions

MISSION: On a separate piece of paper, develop a 100-word response to the following questions.

1. Outline the best approach to losing body fat without hindering your RMR.

2. Explain the different purposes of pre-exercise nutrition, during-exercise nutrition, and post-exercise nutrition.

3. What advice would you give active individuals and athletes to ensure appropriate hydration and rehydration during exercise?

WORKSHEET

My Notes on Chapter 14

Use the space below to make notes on the questions on the facing page, to record any thoughts and ideas you have on this chapter, and to store study tips to help you prepare for tests and exams.

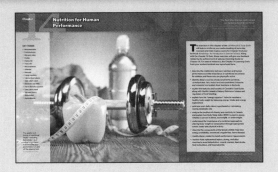

Chapter 14 Review (Student Textbook page 401)

Knowledge

1. Distinguish between macronutrients and micro-nutrients and give several examples of foods that contain one or both of these two categories of nutrients.
2. In a table, list the three main macronutrients, several common food sources for each macronutrient, and the percentage of energy each macronutrient should supply in an average adult's diet.
3. What three factors contribute to our daily caloric need? What might be the easiest lifestyle changes someone could make to tip the energy equation so that energy is not stored as fat?
4. Differentiate between metabolic rate (MR), basal metabolic rate (BMR), and resting metabolic rate (RMR) and list five factors that affect your metabolic rate. Why is knowing your RMR important?
5. State the four general rules for losing body fat without hindering your RMR.
6. Identify the three components of the female athlete triad, and state the underlying cause of this condition.
7. Identify the different goals and strategies related to pre-exercise, during exercise, and post-exercise nutrition and hydration.
8. If you were going to participate in an all-day rugby tournament during a hot, humid day in the summer, how would you plan your fluid intake over the course of the day to prevent poor performance and/or heat-related injuries?

Thinking and Inquiry

9. What is your recommended daily intake for sodium, fibre, and calcium? To find out, go to the Health Canada website and look up the Dietary Reference Intakes (DRI) for your age and gender. With a partner, discuss whether and how you need to modify your intake of these substances.
10. Suppose you have a friend who takes supplemental vitamins and minerals well in excess of recommended levels. Based on what you have learned in this chapter, what advice would you give your friend?
11. Estimate your RMR using (a) the Harris-Benedict equation and (b) the "quick method." How do the values derived from these two methods compare with each other? Which method do you think more closely estimates your RMR, and why? Now estimate your daily caloric need based on your regular activity level. What is the ultimate goal of such calculations?
12. If an active individual (male or female) were unknowingly not taking in enough calories to meet his or her energy needs, what symptoms might signal insufficient energy intake?
13. With a partner, write and exchange a question you would like to ask a vegetarian or vegan athlete about how they meet their nutritional needs, and collaborate on finding an answer to the question.
14. What symptoms and behaviours demonstrated by athletes at an endurance event on a hot day might indicate the need to summon emergency medical personnel? Explain your answer.

Communication

15. Write a blog for the health column of your school newspaper in which you explain why complex carbohydrates are generally better for us compared to simple carbohydrates.
16. You have a friend who announces plans to go on a "crash diet" to lose weight as summer beach weather approaches. Explain to your friend how and why a gradual weight loss program is a healthier choice compared to a "vicious diet cycle."
17. Draw a labelled sketch or use a graphic organizer of your choice to summarize how athletes at every level must modify basic protein, carbohydrate, and fat requirements in order to optimize performance.

Application

18. Bring in a tinned, bottled, or packaged food of your choice and study its nutrition facts label. Based on the information the label provides about the 13 core ingredients contained in the food product, evaluate whether the product is fundamentally healthy or unhealthy and justify your evaluation.
19. Track your food consumption and your levels of physical activity (sedentary, moderately active, or active) for seven days. (a) How does your diet compare to what is recommended for you in Canada's Food Guide? (b) How could you make easy changes to improve your diet based on the guide's recommendations? (c) Based on this one-week record, conclude whether you are achieving a negative energy balance, a stable energy balance, or a positive energy balance.

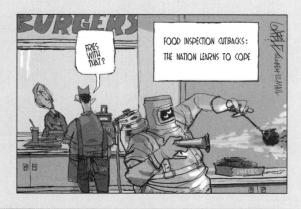

Nutrition experts recommend that no more than 10 percent of our daily caloric intake come from saturated fats, and that we keep all fat intake below 30 percent of our daily caloric intake. (CP Photo/Brian Gable/The Globe and Mail)

Training and Human Performance

KEY TERMS

- F.I.T.T. Principle
- Training principles
- Target Heart Rate (THR)
- One-Repetition Maximum (1RM)
- Periodization
- Flexibility training
- Core training
- Cardiorespiratory training
- Resistance training
- Circuit and stage training
- Plyometrics training
- Speed/agility/quickness training
- Balance training
- Heat exchange
- Health-related fitness
- Performance-related fitness
- CSEP Physical Activity Training for Health (CSEP-PATH)

Hurdler Perdita Felicien in training at the Glenmore Athletic Park in Calgary, Alberta. Felicien attended the University of Illinois on scholarship, where she studied kinesiology.

CP Photo/Jeff McIntosh

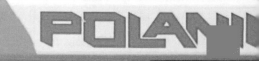

The exercises in this chapter of the *Lab Manual & Study Guide* will help to reinforce your understanding of some key concepts and main topics covered in Chapter 15 of your textbook *Kinesiology: An Introduction to Exercise Science*. Along with the Chapter 15 Quiz, these exercises will give you feedback related to the achievement of selected Learning Goals for Chapter 15. For ease of reference, the Chapter 15 Learning Goals from your student textbook are reproduced here:

- analyze the effects of training on human performance

- explain the F.I.T.T. training principle (Frequency, Intensity, Time, and Type) and training principles that complement it (progressive overload, specificity, reversibility, diminishing returns, and individual differences)

- describe the nature and purpose of various training methods, e.g., periodization, resistance training, plyometrics training, and cardiorespiratory training

- analyze the effects of different environmental conditions and other factors such as rest and recovery or burnout on the body during training and physical activity

- determine training goals that are S.M.A.R.T.: specific, measurable, attainable, realistic, and timely

- identify the stages and components of safe, effective individualized training programs for overall fitness, health-related fitness, and performance-related fitness

- describe the purpose and features of various tools for assessing specific areas of personal fitness, including the CSEP-PATH assessment and other approved tests

- determine factors to consider in designing sample training programs and specialized fitness plans for individuals with varying needs and at varying fitness levels, based on counselling and physiological appraisal (testing)

- describe the role of the trainer in setting fitness goals

WORKSHEET

15.1 Environmental and Other Factors Affecting Training

Environmental factors such as extreme
temperatures (both hot and cold), high
humidity, high altitude, and air quality can have
a significant impact on physical training and
physical performance.

Name: _____

Date: _____

(A) The Effects of Environmental Factors on Training

MISSION: Research how the various environmental factors listed in the left-hand column of the table can have a significant impact on physical training and physical performance, using historical or current sporting events as the basis of your research findings. A sample entry has been included to assist you.

Environmental Factors	Effects on the Body and on Training
High altitude	At the track and field competition in the 1968 Olympic Games in Mexico City, every long-distance event was won in a time significantly slower than the world record. Athletes born and raised at high altitudes dominated; those from sea-level areas attempted to train at altitude to prepare but almost none of their efforts were successful. Athletes in sprints, however, recorded many excellent times due to the "thinner" air.
Cold climates	
Hot climates (with high humidity)	
Air quality	

(B) Other Key Factors Affecting Training

MISSION: Research how the various factors listed in the left-hand column of the table can have a significant impact on physical training and physical performance, using historical or current sporting events as the basis of your research findings. A sample entry has been included to assist you.

Key Factors	Effects on the Body and on Training
Sleep	Starting in 2009, Fatigue Science, a small company based in Vancouver, has supplied the Vancouver Canucks hockey team with watch-like devices called Readibands to assess the quality and quantity of the players' sleep. Data have shown that athletes need more sleep than they think they do. Insufficient sleep reduces reaction time and slows down thinking processes. The Canucks' performance record while on the road has improved since using the Readibands.
Rest	
Recovery	
Avoiding burnout and overtraining	
S.M.A.R.T. goal setting	

WORKSHEET

15.2 Personal Fitness Assessment and Program Design

Assessing your own fitness and wellness levels and adjusting your lifestyle to attain specific goals are important aspects of designing and carrying out a health-related or a performance-related fitness plan.

Name: _____

Date: _____

MISSION: This exercise introduces you to the **Canadian Society for Exercise Physiology (CSEP)** and its certification program for exercise professionals. You will find samples of CSEP-generated questionnaires and fitness assessments that can help you—with appropriate supervision—design your own fitness plan.

First, fill out the **PAR-Q & YOU PHYSICAL ACTIVITY READINESS QUESTIONNAIRE** on page 243 to identify any health-related problems that might require medical attention. (CSEP's PAR-Q+ tool, available on the CSEP website, is designed for individuals who might require even further screening by a medical professional.)

1. Physical Activity and Sedentary Behaviour Questionnaire (PASB-Q)

Complete the **Physical Activity and Sedentary Behaviour Questionnaire (PASB-Q)** on pages 244-245. Note your ranking with respect to the Health Benefits Rating for this assessment and record your score on the Evaluation Summary Report on page 258.

2. Fantastic Lifestyle Checklist

Next, complete the **Fantastic Lifestyle Checklist** on pages 246-247. You may then choose to carry out a series of body composition and fitness assessments (described below), under the supervision of a qualified teacher, coach, or fitness instructor. Note your ranking with respect to the Health Benefits Rating for this assessment and record your score on the Evaluation Summary Report on page 258.

3. Body Composition Assessment

While there are several ways to assess body composition, the CSEP-PATH uses Body Mass Index (BMI) and waist circumference (WC) for adults aged 20-65 years. See "Assessing Body Composition for Clients Under Age 20 Years" on page 251. Note your ranking with respect to the Health Benefits Rating for this assessment and record your score on the Evaluation Summary Report on page 258.

4. Aerobic (Cardiorespiratory) Assessment

For persons aged 15–69 who have no difficulty with balance or coordination and who do not prefer a cycling option, CSEP recommends the Modified Canadian Aerobic Fitness Test (mCAFT). This is a "sub-maximal" assessment, which means that you will not be going "all-out." See a description of this aerobic

fitness test on pages 252-253. Note your ranking with respect to the Health Benefits Rating for this assessment and record your score on the Evaluation Summary Report on page 258.

5. Musculoskeletal Fitness Assessment

The CSEP-PATH assesses muscle strength, power, and endurance, as well as flexibility and balance. The following six musculoskeletal fitness tests are described on pages 254-256: (1) Grip Strength, (2) Push-Up, (3) Sit and Reach,(4) Vertical Jump, (5) Back Extension, and (6) One-leg Stance. Note your ranking with respect to the Health Benefits Rating for this assessment and record your score on the Evaluation Summary Report on page 259.

Interpreting Your Results

Once you have completed the assessments, you can interpret your results by answering the following:

- In which assessment did you achieve your best results?

  _____

- In which assessment did your results show a need for improvement? Why do you think this was so?

  _____
  _____

- With reference to specific components of fitness, how could you improve your overall results?

  _____

Design Your Own Fitness Program

You can now design an exercise program to meet your personal needs. Refer to the sample training programs on page 429 of your textbook and use one of the templates on pages 260-261 of this Study Guide. Apply the F.I.T.T. principle and any other training principles (described in your textbook) to design an eight-week fitness program. Re-take the tests after the eight weeks to determine any improvements.

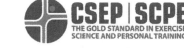

Canadian Society for Exercise Physiology (CSEP)

In North America, two principle affiliated professional associations offer certification programs that acknowledge advanced academic and practical qualification in exercise science, physical activity, fitness, and health. These two associations are the American College of Sports Medicine (ACSM) and the Canadian Society for Exercise Physiology (CSEP).

CSEP is Canada's leading scientific research authority and source of expertise in physical activity, health, fitness, and training. CSEP ensures that Canadians have access to evidence-based physical activity and exercise programming, customized to meet their needs and requirements.

Canadians seeking to become qualified exercise professionals pursue certification options offered by CSEP. CSEP's rigorous, evidence-based certification process is what sets it apart from others.

Two Levels of Certification

CSEP offers two levels of certification based on a candidate's academic background and work experience in the field:

- a **CSEP Certified Personal Trainer® (CSEP-CPT)**, and

- a **CSEP Certified Exercise Physiologist® (CSEP-CEP)** (more advanced than a CSEP-CPT).

Both categories of professionals provide client-centred guidance and advice based on scientific evidence and extensive training, building on the foundation of the Canadian Physical Activity Guidelines (CSEP, 2011), which are listed on page 242.

The CSEP-CPT is certified to administer assessments, including appropriate sub-maximal fitness assessment protocols, to apparently healthy individuals, interpret results, develop a client-centred physical activity action plan, and act as a personal trainer.

The CSEP Certified Exercise Physiologist® (CSEP-CEP) is an advanced certification that includes a broader repertoire of clients and broader assessment and prescription services. A CSEP-CEP must have completed at least a 4-year university degree in Kinesiology, Human Kinetics, or Health Science.

CSEP-CPT Certification

To be certified as a CSEP-CPT, candidates must meet the following requirements:

- ✔ Academic pre-requisites: A minimum of 2 years of College Diploma or University Degree coursework addressing the CPT core competencies (e.g., Anatomy and Physiology; Psychological Characteristics and Motivational Strategies; Theory and Methods of Health-Related Physical Fitness; Physical Activity/Exercise Prescription and Design; Safety and Emergency Procedures; Documentation, Administration and Professionalism);

- ✔ Hold current emergency/standard first aid and CPR Level C;

- ✔ Successfully complete a national theory and practical exam;

- ✔ Participate in continuing education/professional development; and

- ✔ Carry annual CSEP membership including mandatory insurance policy ($3 million professional and commercial liability).

For further information on CSEP and CSEP certification programs, go to **www.csep.ca**. You can also sign up for a free e-newsletter and follow CSEP updates on Facebook and Twitter.

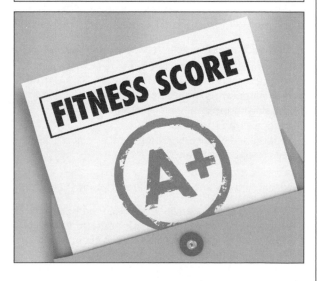

The physical activity, fitness, and lifestyle assessment administered by a CSEP-CPT is exclusively that outlined in the CSEP Physical Activity Training for Health (CSEP-PATH) Resource Manual. The assessment provides information to help clients safely and effectively build regular physical activity into their daily lives to improve their health and well-being.

The CSEP-PATH itself is a five-step sequence based on the 5As: Ask, Assess, Advise, Agree, and Assist/ Arrange. The CSEP-PATH helps clients set realistic goals and devise action plans for achieving them. For each CSEP-PATH step, key "best practices" in guiding individuals to health-related behaviour change are accompanied by relevant evidence-based tools.

The CSEP-PATH evaluates physical activity, sedentary behaviour, and other lifestyle factors (e.g., nutrition and alcohol use) by means of simple questionnaires.

CSEP Fitness Assessment Protocols

The fitness assessment involves a series of physical tests and measurements. Some of these (e.g., height, body weight, and waist circumference) require no physical exertion. Those that evaluate aerobic and musculoskeletal fitness require physical exertion and are outlined briefly below. All clients sign an Informed Consent Form prior to proceeding with the tests.

- Aerobic Fitness Assessment Measures
  Aerobic fitness is estimated based on heart rate response to one of four sub-maximal protocols, depending on the client's interests and capabilities: a multi-stage step test, single-stage treadmill walking, a one-mile walk, or a multi-stage cycle test. Post-exercise heart rate and blood pressure are monitored after the respective protocol before proceeding to other measures to ensure an appropriate recovery.

- Musculoskeletal Fitness Assessment Measures
  Six simple tests are performed to evaluate musculoskeletal fitness: grip strength (strength of hands, forearms); push-up (endurance of chest, shoulders, arms); sit and reach (flexibility of hips); vertical jump (power of legs); back extension (endurance of back); one-leg stance (balance and leg strength/endurance).

Physical Activity and Exercise Prescription

A CSEP-CPT employs evidence-based methods and tools to prescribe specific intensity, duration, and frequency of physical activity for each client. (This does not include maximal effort aerobic physical activity or muscle and bone strengthening exercise.)

Canadian Physical Activity Guidelines

The client-centred physical activity action plans based on CSEP-PATH assessment results build on the foundation of the Canadian Physical Activity Guidelines (CSEP, 2011), as follows:

Adults aged 18-64 years should accumulate at least 150 minutes of moderate- to vigorous-intensity aerobic physical activity per week, in bouts of 10 minutes or more. It is also beneficial to add muscle and bone strengthening activities using major muscle groups, at least 2 days per week. More daily physical activity provides greater health benefits.

Adults aged 65 years and older should accumulate at least 150 minutes of moderate- to vigorous-intensity aerobic physical activity per week, in bouts of 10 minutes or more. It is also beneficial to add muscle and bone strengthening activities using major muscle groups, at least 2 days per week.

Adults aged 65 years and older who have poor mobility should perform physical activities to enhance balance and prevent falls. More daily physical activity provides greater health benefits.

Children aged 5-11 years and youth aged 12-17 years should accumulate at least 60 minutes of moderate- to vigorous-intensity physical activity daily. This should include: vigorous-intensity activities at least 3 days per week; and activities that strengthen muscle and bone at least 3 days per week. More daily physical activity provides greater health benefits.

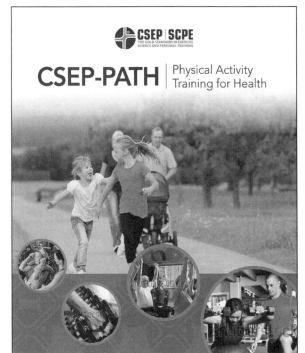

Courtesy of the Canadian Society for Exercise Physiology.

Physical Activity Readiness
Questionnaire - PAR-Q
(revised 2002)

PAR-Q & YOU

(A Questionnaire for People Aged 15 to 69)

Regular physical activity is fun and healthy, and increasingly more people are starting to become more active every day. Being more active is very safe for most people. However, some people should check with their doctor before they start becoming much more physically active.

If you are planning to become much more physically active than you are now, start by answering the seven questions in the box below. If you are between the ages of 15 and 69, the PAR-Q will tell you if you should check with your doctor before you start. If you are over 69 years of age, and you are not used to being very active, check with your doctor.

Common sense is your best guide when you answer these questions. Please read the questions carefully and answer each one honestly: check YES or NO.

YES	NO		
☐	☐	1.	Has your doctor ever said that you have a heart condition <u>and</u> that you should only do physical activity recommended by a doctor?
☐	☐	2.	Do you feel pain in your chest when you do physical activity?
☐	☐	3.	In the past month, have you had chest pain when you were not doing physical activity?
☐	☐	4.	Do you lose your balance because of dizziness or do you ever lose consciousness?
☐	☐	5.	Do you have a bone or joint problem (for example, back, knee or hip) that could be made worse by a change in your physical activity?
☐	☐	6.	Is your doctor currently prescribing drugs (for example, water pills) for your blood pressure or heart condition?
☐	☐	7.	Do you know of <u>any other reason</u> why you should not do physical activity?

If you answered

YES to one or more questions

Talk with your doctor by phone or in person BEFORE you start becoming much more physically active or BEFORE you have a fitness appraisal. Tell your doctor about the PAR-Q and which questions you answered YES.

- You may be able to do any activity you want — as long as you start slowly and build up gradually. Or, you may need to restrict your activities to those which are safe for you. Talk with your doctor about the kinds of activities you wish to participate in and follow his/her advice.
- Find out which community programs are safe and helpful for you.

NO to all questions

If you answered NO honestly to <u>all</u> PAR-Q questions, you can be reasonably sure that you can:
- start becoming much more physically active — begin slowly and build up gradually. This is the safest and easiest way to go.
- take part in a fitness appraisal — this is an excellent way to determine your basic fitness so that you can plan the best way for you to live actively. It is also highly recommended that you have your blood pressure evaluated. If your reading is over 144/94, talk with your doctor before you start becoming much more physically active.

DELAY BECOMING MUCH MORE ACTIVE:
- if you are not feeling well because of a temporary illness such as a cold or a fever — wait until you feel better; or
- if you are or may be pregnant — talk to your doctor before you start becoming more active.

PLEASE NOTE: If your health changes so that you then answer YES to any of the above questions, tell your fitness or health professional. Ask whether you should change your physical activity plan.

<u>Informed Use of the PAR-Q</u>: The Canadian Society for Exercise Physiology, Health Canada, and their agents assume no liability for persons who undertake physical activity, and if in doubt after completing this questionnaire, consult your doctor prior to physical activity.

No changes permitted. You are encouraged to photocopy the PAR-Q but only if you use the entire form.

NOTE: If the PAR-Q is being given to a person before he or she participates in a physical activity program or a fitness appraisal, this section may be used for legal or administrative purposes.

"I have read, understood and completed this questionnaire. Any questions I had were answered to my full satisfaction."

NAME _____

SIGNATURE _____ DATE_____

SIGNATURE OF PARENT _____ WITNESS _____
or GUARDIAN (for participants under the age of majority)

Note: This physical activity clearance is valid for a maximum of 12 months from the date it is completed and becomes invalid if your condition changes so that you would answer YES to any of the seven questions.

CSEP | SCPE
THE WORLD STANDARD INTEGRATED SCIENCE AND PERSONAL TRAINING

© Canadian Society for Exercise Physiology www.csep.ca/forms

Source: CSEP-PATH Physical Activity Training for Health Resource Manual, 2013. Reprinted with permission from the Canadian Society for Exercise Physiology.

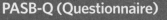

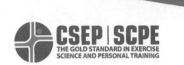

CSEP-PATH: PHYSICAL ACTIVITY AND SEDENTARY BEHAVIOUR QUESTIONNAIRE (PASB-Q) YOUTH (12 - 17 YEARS)

Please answer the following questions based on what you do in a typical week. To increase accuracy, you may wish to log your physical activity and sedentary behavior for one week prior to answering the questions.

Aerobic Physical Activity

1. Frequency: In a typical week, how many days do you do moderate-intensity (like biking) to vigorous-intensity (like running) aerobic physical activity?

    _____ days/week

2. Time or Duration: On average for days that you at least moderate-intensity aerobic physical activity (as specified above), how many minutes do you do?

    _____ minutes/day

3. In a typical week, how many days do you do vigorous-intensity aerobic physical activity?

    _____ days/week

Muscle Strengthening Physical Activity

4. Frequency: In a typical week, how many times do you do muscle strengthening activities (such as resistance training, wall climbing, or competitive sport)?

    _____ times/week

5. Time or Duration: On average for days that you do muscle strengthening activities (as specified above), how many minutes do you do?

    _____ minutes/week

Total Physical Activity (add responses to questions 2 and 5) _____ minutes/day

Perceived Aerobic Fitness

6. In general, would you say that your aerobic fitness (ability to walk/run distances) is:

____ Excellent   ____ Very Good   ____ Good   ____ Fair   ____ Poor

Sedentary Behaviour

7. On a typical day, how many hours do you spend in continuous sitting: at school, work, volunteer commitments and commuting (i.e., by motorized transport)?

☐ None   ☐ < 1 hour   ☐ 1 to < 2   ☐ 2 to < 3

☐ 3 to < 4   ☐ 4 to < 5   ☐ 5 to < 6   ☐ > 6

8. On a typical day, how many hours do you watch television, use a computer, play video games, read, and spend sitting quietly during your leisure time?

☐ None   ☐ < 1 hour   ☐ 1 to < 2

☐ 3 to < 4   ☐ 4 to < 5   ☐ 5 to < 6

Total Sedentary Behaviour (add responses to questions 7 and 8) ____ hours/day

9. When sitting for prolonged periods (one hour or more), at what time interval would you typically take a break to stand and move around for two minutes?

☐ < 10 minutes

☐ 10 to < 20 minutes

☐ 20 to < 30 minutes

☐ 30 to < 45 minutes

☐ 45 to < 1 hour

☐ 1 to < 1.5 hours

☐ 1.5 to < 2 hours

☐ > 2 hours

Converting the PASB-Q Results to Health Benefit Ratings—Youth (12-17 Years)					
Health Benefit Rating	Total Physical Activity (Min/Day)	Vigorous Aerobic Physical Activity (Times/Week)	Strength Physical Activity (Times/Week)	Perceived Aerobic Fitness	Sedentary Behaviour (Hours/Day)
Excellent	120+	6+	6+	Excellent	<2
Very Good	90-119	4-5	4-5	Very Good	2-4
Good	60-89	3	3	Good	4-6
Fair	30-59	1-2	1-2	Fair	6-8
Poor	0-29	0	0	Poor	>8

Source: CSEP-PATH Physical Activity Training for Health Resource Manual, 2013. Reprinted with permission from the Canadian Society for Exercise Physiology.

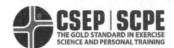

FANTASTIC LIFESTYLE CHECKLIST

Place an 'X' beside the box which best describes your behaviour over the last couple of weeks. Explanations of questions and scoring are provided on the next page.

FAMILY FRIENDS	I have someone to talk to about things that are important to me	almost never	seldom	some of the time	fairly often	almost always
	I give and receive affection	almost never	seldom	some of the time	fairly often	almost always
ACTIVITY	I am vigorously active for at least 30 minutes per day e.g., running, cycling, etc	less than once/week	1-2 times/ week	3 times/ week	4 times/ week	5 or more times/ week
	I am moderately active (gardening, climbing stairs, walking, housework)	less than once/week	1-2 times/ week	3 times/ week	4 times/ week	5 or more times/ week
NUTRITION	I eat a balanced diet (see explanation)	almost never	seldom	some of the time	fairly often	almost always
	I often eat excess 1) sugar, or 2) salt, or 3) animal fats, or 4) junk food	four of these	three of these	two of these	one of these	none of these
	I am within _____kg of my healthy weight	not within 8 kg	8 kg (20 lbs)	6 kg (15 lbs)	4 kg (10 lbs)	2 kg (5 lbs)
TOBACCO TOXICS	I smoke tobacco	more than 10 times/ week	1 – 10 times/ week	none in the past 6 months	none in the past year	none in the past 5 years
	I use drugs such as marijuana, cocaine	sometimes				never
	I overuse prescribed or 'over the counter' drugs	almost daily	fairly often	only occasionally	almost never	never
	I drink caffeine-containing coffee, tea or cola	more than 10/day	7-10/ day	3-6/day	1-2/day	never

Category	Statement	more than 20 drinks	13-20 drinks	11-12 drinks	8-10 drinks	0-7 drinks
ALCOHOL	My average alcohol intake per week is _____ (see explanation)	more than 20 drinks	13-20 drinks	11-12 drinks	8-10 drinks	0-7 drinks
	I drink more than four drinks on an occasion	almost daily	fairly often	only occasionally	almost never	never
	I drive after drinking	sometimes				never
SLEEP SEATBELT STRESS SAFE SEX	I sleep well and feel rested	almost never	seldom	some of the time	fairly often	almost always
	I use seatbelts	never	seldom	some of the time	most of the time	always
	I am able to cope with the stresses in my life	almost never	seldom	some of the time	fairly often	almost always
	I relax and enjoy leisure time	almost never	seldom	some of the time	fairly often	almost always
	I practice safe sex (see explanation)	almost never	seldom	some of the time	fairly often	almost always
TYPE OF BEHAVIOUR	I seem to be in a hurry	almost always	fairly often	some of the time	seldom	almost never
	I feel angry or hostile	almost always	fairly often	some of the time	seldom	almost never
INSIGHT	I am a positive or optimistic thinker	almost never	seldom	some of the time	fairly often	almost always
	I feel tense or uptight	almost always	fairly often	some of the time	seldom	almost never
	I feel sad or depressed	almost always	fairly often	some of the time	seldom	almost never
CAREER	I am satisfied with my job or role	almost never	seldom	some of the time	fairly often	almost always
STEP 1	Total the X's in each column	→				
STEP 2	Multiply the totals by The numbers indicated (write your answer in the box below)	→ o	x 1	x 2	x 3	x 4
STEP 3	Add your scores across The bottom for your					
	Grand total	→ o				=

Source: CSEP-PATH Physical Activity Training for Health Resource Manual, 2013. Reprinted with permission from the Canadian Society for Exercise Physiology.

▼ A BALANCED DIET

According to Canada's Food Guide, different people need different amounts of food. The amount of food you need every day from the 4 food groups and other foods depends on your age, body size, activity level, whether you are male or female and if your are pregnant or breast feeding. That's why the Food Guide gives a lower and higher number of servings for each food group. For example, young children can choose the lower number of servings, and male teenagers can select the higher number. Most other people can choose servings somewhere in between. The ranges below are for adult men and women from 19 to 50+.

Grain Products	Vegetables & Fruit	Milk Products	Meat & Alternatives	Other Foods
Choose whole grain and enriched products more often	Choose dark green and orange vegetables more often	Choose lower fat milk products more often	Choose leaner meats, poultry and fish, as well as dried peas, beans and lentils more often	Taste and enjoyment can also come from other foods and beverages that are not part of the 4 food groups. Some of these are higher in fat or calories, so use these foods in moderation.

Recommended number of servings per day

Grain Products	Vegetables & Fruit	Milk Products	Meat & Alternatives	Other Foods
6 - 8	7 - 10	2 - 3	2 - 3	

▼ ALCOHOL INTAKE

1 drink equals:		Canadian	Metric	U.S.
1 bottle of beer	5% alcohol	12 oz.	340.8 ml	10 oz.
1 glass wine	12% alcohol	5 oz.	142 ml	4.5 oz.
1 shot spirits	40% alcohol	1.5 oz.	42.6 ml	1.25 oz.

▼ SAFE SEX

Refers to the use of methods of preventing infection or conception

WHAT DOES THE SCORE MEAN?

→

85-100	70-84	55-69	35-54	0-34
EXCELLENT	VERY GOOD	GOOD	FAIR	NEEDS IMPROVEMENT

NOTE: A low total score does not mean that you have failed. There is always the chance to change your lifestyle – starting now. Look at the areas where you scored a 0 or 1 and decide which areas you want to work on first.

TIPS:

1. Don't try to change all the areas at once. This will be too overwhelming for you.

2. Writing down your proposed changes and your overall goal will help you to succeed.

3. Make changes in small steps towards the overall goal.

4. Enlist the help of a friend to make similar changes and/or to support you in your attempts.

5. Congratulate yourself for achieving each step. Give yourself appropriate rewards.

6. Ask your physical activity professional (CSEP-Qualified Exercise Professional), family physician, nurse or health department for more information on any of these areas.

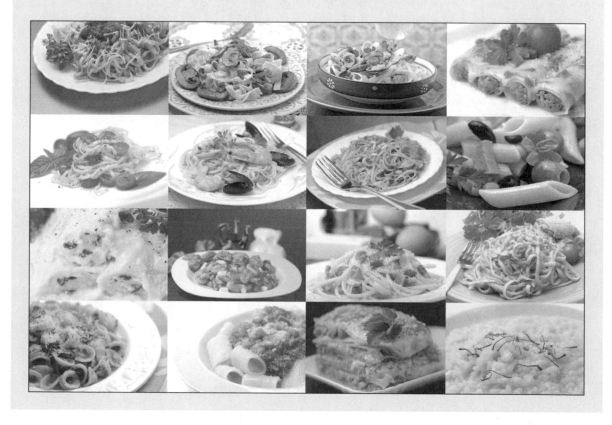

Source: CSEP-PATH Physical Activity Training for Health Resource Manual, 2013. Reprinted with permission from the Canadian Society for Exercise Physiology. Photo courtesy of Marzia Giacobbe/Shutterstock

Assessing body weight and body fat distribution is important, as excess body fat (particularly when located around the abdomen) signals increased risk of a variety of health problems, including type 2 diabetes, hypertension, dyslipidemia, coronary artery disease, stroke, osteoarthritis and certain forms of cancer.

While there are several ways to assess body composition, the CSEP-PATH uses **Body Mass Index (BMI)** and **waist circumference (WC)**. Together, the BMI and WC provide a more robust estimate of health benefit/risk associated with body fatness and fat distribution than any single measure on its own. However, when assessing body composition for youth aged under 20 years, the CSEP-PATH recommends using BMI alone, while taking into account age and gender variations as well, as explained on the following page.

Body Mass Index (BMI)

BMI is an indirect measure of body fatness, which is correlated with health risk and is a predictor of mortality at the population level (i.e., increased risk among underweight, overweight, and obese individuals). However, BMI does not distinguish between fat mass and fat-free mass, and provides no information on the distribution of body fat.

The correlation between BMI and body fatness can vary by gender and age (e.g., at the same BMI, women tend to have more body fat than men, and older people tend to have more body fat than younger individuals). As well, trained athletes may have a higher BMI (i.e., in the overweight category) because of increased muscularity rather than body fatness. In non-athletes, a BMI of 30 or more is considered a very reliable indicator of obesity. (Lau et al., 2007)

Calculating BMI

BMI gives a rough indication as to whether your body weight (mass) is appropriate for your height. To find your BMI, follow these steps:

- Using a tape measure (or fixed-height wall chart), find your height in metres (m).

- Using a weighing scale, find your weight in kilograms (kg).

- To calculate your BMI, divide your weight in kilograms by your height in metres squared (m²).

$$BMI = \frac{w}{m^2}$$

The male below is 1.68 m tall and weighs 83.5 kg. His BMI is 29.6. This value has been calculated by dividing 83.5 by 1.68 x 1.68 (his height in metres squared).

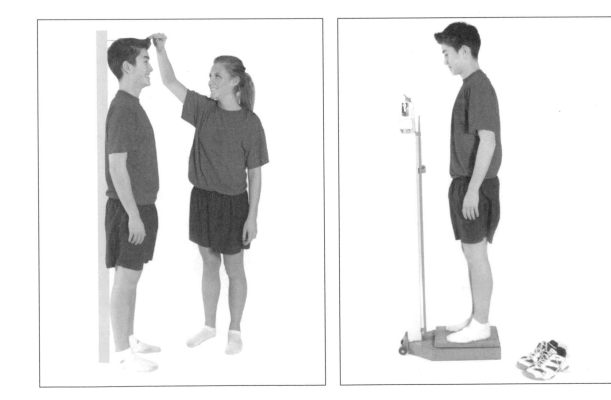

Assessing Body Composition for Clients under 20 Years of Age

For clients under 20 years old, the World Health Organization's **BMI-for-age growth charts** are used to assess risk of overweight and underweight (WHO Child Growth Standards, 2006). Because BMI changes substantially as children get older, and because adiposity varies with age and gender during childhood and adolescence, BMI is age- and gender-specific. The growth charts for boys and girls aged 5 to 19 years are shown below.

The charts show the distribution (percentiles) of BMI results for a representative sample of boys and girls. When assessing BMI results for youth under 20 years, qualified exercise professionals will be able to locate the BMI on the relevant chart and classify the client according to the table below.

For example, a boy aged 15 years, weighing 80 kg and measuring 170 cm in height would have a BMI of $80/1.7^2 = 27.7$. The chart for boys places him above the 97th percentile. He is rated as Obese. Full-sized charts are available through the Dietitians of Canada website (www.dieticians.ca) and many other online sources.

BMI Categories for Children and Youth		
BMI Category	**Age 2-5 years**	**Age 5-19 Years**
Severely thin	< 1st percentile	< 1st percentile
Thin	< 3rd percentile	< 3rd percentile
Risk of overweight	> 85th percentile	--
Overweight	> 97th percentile	> 85th percentile
Obese	> 99.9th percentile	> 97th percentile
Severely obese	--	> 99.9th percentile

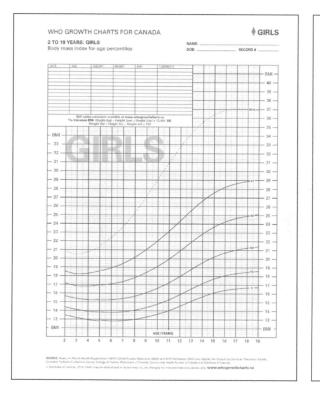

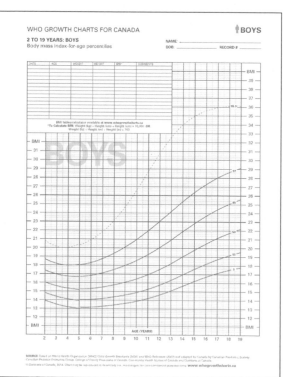

Cardiorespiratory (or aerobic) fitness is one of the most important determinants of health. It reflects the efficiency of an individual's heart, lungs, and blood vessels in transporting oxygen to working muscles, and the muscles' ability to use that oxygen to do work. As such, it refers to an individual's ability to sustain physical effort over a period of time (e.g., walking, running, biking, climbing, swimming) and ability to respond to emergencies.

The CSEP-PATH provides four different protocols to estimate aerobic fitness, as summarized in the table below. Each of the aerobic fitness tests has common termination criteria and recovery procedures. For example, an aerobic fitness test will end if and when the client reaches the "Ceiling Heart Rate" (85% of 220-age) or shows signs of physiological distress.

The Modified Canadian Aerobic Fitness Test (mCAFT) is outlined on the following page. CSEP recommends that a heart rate monitor be used during this assessment.

CSEP-PATH Aerobic Fitness Test Protocols			
Protocol	**Description**	**Suitable For**	**Time Requirement**
mCAFT	Multi-stage step test	15-69 years	15-20 minutes
Treadmill Walking Test	Single-stage treadmill walking (5% grade)	Sedentary adults (20-59 years)	15-20 minutes
One-Mile Walk	Brisk walking over 1 mile flat measured distance	Sedentary and/or older adults (20-69 years) who may prefer a walking prescription	25-35 minutes
Cycle Ergometer Test	Multi-stage cycle test	Clients aged 15-69 years who have difficulty with balance or coordination and/or prefer a cycling prescription	20-30 minutes

mCAFT (Two-Step Variation)

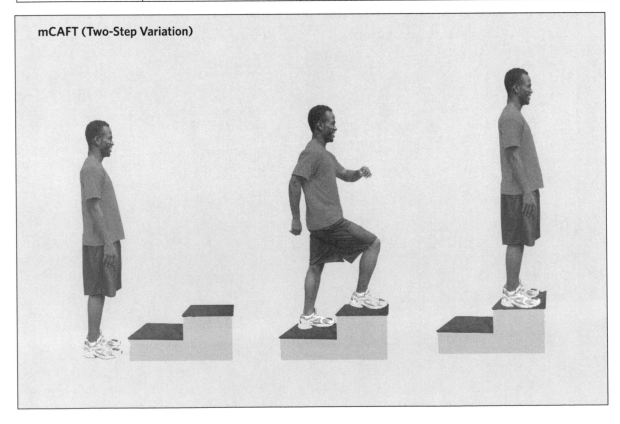

The Modified Canadian Aerobic Fitness Test (mCAFT)

The **mCAFT** is a multi-stage, sub-maximal test to estimate VO_2 max for clients aged 15-69 years. A qualified exercise professional first demonstrates the procedure and has the client practise it both without and with the pre-recorded music that sets the pace, or "cadence" (steps per minute) for the test.

Everyone begins with a 2-step sequence; some may complete the assessment with a single-step sequence using a higher step. For persons aged 15-19, the starting stage cadence is 3 for females and 4 for males (see the table below).

Cued by the music, the client steps up and down on a platform at predetermined speeds based on their age and gender. The client stops stepping and remains motionless when the music stops at the end of each 3-minute stage, whereupon their heart rate (HR) is measured for 10 seconds and recorded.

The client completes one or more sessions of three minutes of stepping until they reach their predetermined ceiling heart rate for their age group (85% of the maximal heart rate for that age group). Clients stop once they reach their ceiling heart rate and do not proceed to the next stage.

Calculating VO₂max

Depending on the stage reached, **O_2 cost** can be determined from the first table below. When the test is complete, the client's estimated **VO₂max** can then be calculated using the formula below.

The VO₂max score and the associated Health Benefit Rating (see the second table below) are recorded on the Client Information Sheet.

Always undergo the mCAFT under appropriate supervision. Ensure that you practise the stepping motion so that both feet end up on the top step with legs extended, and your back straight. Ensure that you can maintain a constant stepping tempo.

Additionally, practise finding your heart rate within the window of time allowed on the mCAFT recording.

Most importantly, be sure to review all safety guidelines with the person administering the test before undertaking the assessment.

If you have any concerns as to whether or not you should undertake the mCAFT assessment, consult with your Physical Education teacher and/or your family doctor beforehand.

$$\textbf{85\% HRmax} = 0.85 \,(220 - age)$$
$$\textbf{Estimated VO}_2\textbf{max} = [17.2 + (1.29 \times (O_2Cost) - (0.09 \times wt.\ in\ kg) - (0.18 \times age\ in\ years)]$$

mCAFT Stepping Cadence and O₂ Cost

| Stage | Females | | Males | |
	Cadence	O₂ Cost ($mL \cdot kg^{-1} \cdot min^{-1}$)	Cadence	O₂ Cost ($mL \cdot kg^{-1} \cdot min^{-1}$)
1	66	15.9	66	15.9
2	84	18.0	84	18.0
3	102	22.0	102	22.0
4	114	24.5	114	24.5
5	120	26.3	132	29.5
6	132	29.5	144	33.6
7	144	33.6	118*	36.2
8	118*	36.2	132*	40.1

* One-step procedure.

Estimated VO₂max—Health Benefit Rating (Ages 15–19)

	Males	Females
Excellent	57.4+	49.0+
Very Good	52.4–57.3	43.7–48.9
Good	48.8–52.3	39.5–43.6
Fair	43.6–48.7	36.8–39.4
Needs improvement	<43.6	<36.8

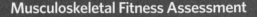

5 Musculoskeletal Fitness Assessment

Musculoskeletal fitness refers to muscles and bones working well together to produce movement. Enhanced musculoskeletal fitness is positively associated with mobility, bone health, psychological well-being, and overall quality of life. Musculoskeletal fitness assessment gives insights into a client's capacity to perform daily activities, cope with emergencies, avoid injury and disability, and maintain functional independence as they age.

The CSEP-PATH assesses muscle strength, power, and endurance, as well as flexibility and balance. An overview of each of the six standardized tests is presented below. A certified CSEP professional follows explicit and detailed instructions in the CSEP-PATH Resource Manual when carrying out these tests with a client.

1. Grip Strength

A hand dynamometer is held in-line with the forearm at the level of the thigh, away from the body. The client squeezes maximally on the dynamometer to exert maximum force. He or she exhales while squeezing. Neither the hand nor the dynamometer should touch the body or any other object.

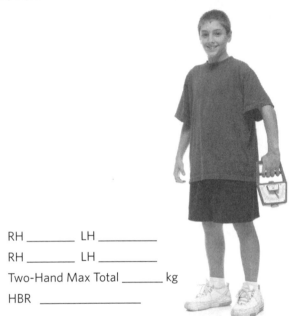

A certified exercise professional measures each hand twice, alternating hands, records the maximum scores for each hand to the nearest kilogram, and combines the maximum scores from each of the left and right hands. The trainer records the results and the associated Health Benefit Rating (see the table on page 261) on a Client Information Sheet. (If you take this test with appropriate supervision, circle the best score from each hand and add them together as the Two-Hand Max Total. Refer to the table on page 257, find your rating, and record it beside "HBR" on the right.)

RH _____   LH _____

RH _____   LH _____

Two-Hand Max Total _____ kg

HBR _____

2. Push-Up

Advise the client to perform as many consecutive push-ups as they can (no time limit). Have clients practise 1-2 repetitions to check for proper technique before beginning. The client lies face down on the mat with legs together, hands pointing forward and positioned under the shoulders. Push up by fulling extending the arms. Keep elbows out from the side. Men use the toes as the pivot point. Women use their knees as the pivot point, keeping their lower legs, ankles, and feet (plantar flexed) in contact with the mat.

For both men and women, the upper body must be kept in a straight line, returning to the starting position with chin to the mat. Stomach and thighs do not touch the mat. (Incorrect repetitions do not count.)

Stop the test if a client feels any pain or discomfort, appears to strain forcibly, or cannot maintain the proper push-up technique over two consecutive repetitions. Advise the client to exhale during the upward phase of the push-up and to avoid holding his/her breath.

A certified exercise professional records the client's total number of push-ups and associated Health Benefit Rating (see the table on page 263) on a Client Information Sheet. (If you take this test with appropriate supervision, record your results below along with your Health Benefit Rating, which you can find in the table on page 257.)

Number of push-ups completed _____

HBR _____

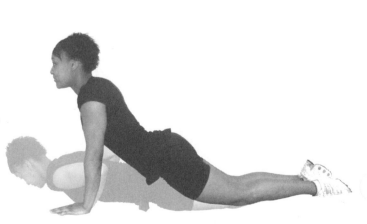

254 ◆ Chapter 15. Training and Human Performance

3. Sit and Reach

This test is the most common way to measure hamstring and lower back flexibility. It is also regarded as a valid and reliable measure of general flexibility.

The client warms up by performing slow stretching using the modified hurdler stretch held for 20 seconds twice on each leg, alternating legs. Without shoes, the client sits with legs fully extended and the soles of the feet placed flat against the flexometer, which should be adjusted so that the balls of the feet rest against the upper crossboards, as shown in the photograph. (The feet must not extend beyond the crossboards.)

A certified exercise professional measures to ensure the inner edge of the feet are 15.24 cm (6 in.) apart. With legs fully extended, arms evenly stretched, palms down and hands together (one over the other), the client bends and reaches forward to push the sliding marker forward along the scale with the fingertips as far as possible, while exhaling. The position of maximum flexion is held for about 2 seconds.

If the knees bend, the trial is not counted. The knees should not be held down and the client should not use a bouncing or a jerking motion. The test is done twice.

Both readings are recorded to the nearest 0.5 cm on the Client Information Sheet and the highest score is used to determine the Health Benefit Rating.

If you take this test under appropriate supervision, use the table on page 257 to determine your Health Benefit Rating (HBR).

Trial 1 _____ cm

Trial 2 _____ cm

HBR _____

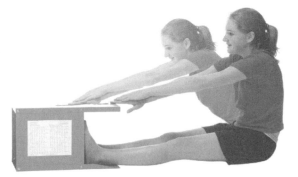

4. Vertical Jump

The client stands sideways to a wall on which a measuring tape has been placed. With feet flat on the floor, the client reaches as high as possible. A certified exercise professional records this beginning height.

Next, the client assumes a ready position with his/her body at a safe distance from the wall. The client moves into a semi-squat position (a run-up or pre-jump is not permitted) and jumps as high as possible, touching the tape at the peak height of the jump. A certified exercise professional records this height.

The client completes this test three times and the highest jump is recorded on the results sheet. A rest of 10–15 seconds occurs between each trial. To determine height jumped, subtract the beginning height from the peak height.

Peak Leg Power. The formula below is used to determine leg power in watts (W). The table on page 257 shows the associated Health Benefit Rating.

Peak Leg Power (W) =

[60.7 × jump height (cm)] +

[45.3 × body mass (kg)] – 2055

= _____ watts

HBR _____

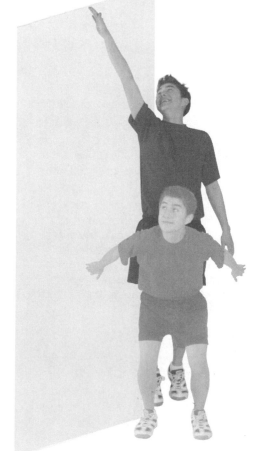

5. Back Extension

This test is a measure of the isometric endurance of the trunk extensor muscles.

Pre-Screening Requirement

This test is not suitable for clients with current back discomfort or pain. Ask the client to lie face down and perform a single straight-leg extension with each leg, followed by the same straight-leg extensions combined with an extension of the opposite arm. If there is discomfort or pain, the test should not be done.

The client lies face down on a mat with the iliac crest positioned at the edge of the platform and the hips, shoulders, and head aligned. The client's lower torso is secured by holding the lower thighs or upper calves.

Prior to initiating the test, the client can support his/her upper body by placing the outstretched hands on the floor. Once the client is secured, they raise and cross their arms on the chest, then maintain the horizontal position with no rotation or lateral shifting for as long as possible, while breathing normally, to a maximum of 3 min (180 s) according to a stopwatch.

Terminate the test if the client experiences pain/discomfort/fatigue, or if their torso drops below the horizontal (allow for one warning and adjustment).

After the test, the client lies on their back with both knees bent for one minute to relax the back muscles.

The certified exercise professional records the number of seconds the horizontal position is maintained and records the associated Health Benefit Rating on the Client Information Sheet.

If you take this test with a qualified exercise professional, record your time and refer to the table on page 257 to find your Health Benefit Rating (HBR).

Note: If you experience any discomfort or pain during the pre-screening test, do not perform the back extension assessment.

Time _____

HBR _____

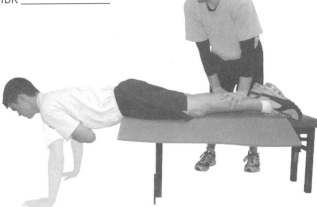

6. One-leg Stance

The client stands barefoot behind or beside a sturdy chair with hands on opposite shoulders crossed in front of the chest. The floor surface should be flat and stable.

With eyes open, the client stands on the leg of their choice, lifting the other foot so that it is near but not touching the ankle of the standing leg. The client holds this position for up to 45 seconds.

Time commences when the client raises the foot. Time ends when: 1) arms are moved (e.g., uncrossed); 2) the raised foot is moved towards or away from the standing limb or touches the floor; 3) the weight-bearing foot is moved to maintain balance; or 4) a maximum of 45 seconds has elapsed. The time is recorded with a stopwatch. The eyes-open test is repeated using the other leg.

The same test is administered with eyes closed, again using alternate legs and the same criteria. If the client loses balance during the first 3 seconds of the eyes-closed test, allow a second try to account for any set-up error. The time for all trials is recorded.

The best times for each of the eyes-open and eyes-closed tests are compared to means by age group and gender in the table at the bottom of page 257.

Perform the test on one leg with eyes open and then with eyes closed. Then repeat the test standing on the other leg.

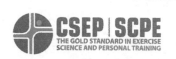

Musculoskeletal Fitness—Health Benefit Ratings

Age (years)	Grip Strength (kg) Male	Grip Strength (kg) Female	Push-ups (#) Male	Push-ups (#) Female	Sit and Reach (cm) Male	Sit and Reach (cm) Female	Vertical Jump (watts) Male	Vertical Jump (watts) Female	Back Extension Male	Back Extension Female
15 - 19										
Excellent	≥ 108	≥ 68	≥ 39	≥ 33	≥ 39	≥ 43	≥ 4644	≥ 3167	158-180	169-180
Very Good	98-107	60-67	29-38	25-32	34-38	38-42	4185-4643	2795-3166	135-157	141-168
Good	90-97	53-59	23-28	18-24	29-33	34-37	3858-4184	2399-2794	119-134	122-140
Fair	79-89	48-52	18-22	12-17	24-28	29-33	3323-3857	2156-2398	91-118	91-121
Poor	≤ 78	≤ 47	≤ 17	≤11	≤ 23	≤ 28	≤ 3322	≤ 2155	≤ 90	≤90
20 - 29										
Excellent	≥115	≥ 70	≥ 36	≥ 30	≥ 40	≥ 41	≥5094	≥ 3250	176-180	180
Very Good	104-114	63-69	29-35	21-29	34-39	37-40	4640-5093	2804-3249	133-175	136-179
Good	95-103	58-62	22-28	15-20	30-33	33-36	4297-4639	2478-2803	99-132	102-135
Fair	84-94	52-57	17-21	10-14	25-29	28-32	3775-4296	2271-2477	86-98	66-101
Poor	≤83	≤51	≤16	≤9	≤24	≤27	≤ 3774	≤ 2270	≤ 85	≤65
30 - 39										
Excellent	≤ 115	≥ 71	≥ 30	≥ 27	≥ 38	≥ 41	≥ 4860	≥ 3193	147-180	180
Very Good	104-114	63-70	22-29	20-26	33-37	36-40	4389-4859	2550-3192	109-146	141-179
Good	95-103	58-62	17-21	13-19	28-32	32-35	3967-4388	2335-2549	91-108	112-140
Fair	84-94	51-57	12-16	8-12	23-27	27-31	3485-3966	2147-2334	86-90	61-111
Poor	≤ 83	≤ 50	≤ 11	≤ 7	≤ 22	≤ 26	≤ 3484	≤ 2146	≤ 55	≤ 60
40 - 49										
Excellent	≥ 108	≥ 69	≥ 25	≥ 24	≥ 35	≥ 38	≥ 4320	≥ 2675	130-180	180
Very Good	97-107	61-68	17-24	15-23	29-34	34-37	3700-4319	2288-2674	84-129	115-179
Good	88-96	54-60	13-16	11-14	24-28	30-33	3242-3699	2101-2287	71-83	80-114
Fair	80-87	49-53	10-12	5-10	18-23	25-29	2708-3241	1688-2100	32-70	42-79
Poor	≤ 79	≤ 48	≤ 9	≤ 4	≤ 17	≤ 24	≤ 2707	≤ 1687	≤ 31	≤ 41
50 - 59										
Excellent	≥ 101	≥ 61	≥ 21	≥ 21	≥ 35	≥ 39	≥ 4019	≥ 2559	120-180	110-180
Very Good	92-100	54-60	13-20	11-20	28-34	33-38	3567-4018	2161-2558	88-119	75-109
Good	84-91	49-53	10-12	7-10	24-27	30-32	2937-3566	1701-2160	54-87	47-74
Fair	76-83	45-48	7-9	2-6	16-23	25-29	2512-2936	1386-1700	20-53	15-46
Poor	≤ 75	≤ 44	≤ 6	≤ 1	≤ 15	≤ 24	≤ 2511	≤ 1385	≤ 19	≤ 14
60 - 69										
Excellent	≥ 100	≥ 54	≥ 18	≥ 17	≥ 33	≥ 35	≥ 3764	≥ 2475	≥ 117	91-180
Very Good	91-99	48-53	11-17	12-16	25-32	31-34	3291-3763	1718-2474	78-116	40-90
Good	84-90	45-47	8-10	5-11	20-24	27-30	2843-3290	1317-1717	52-77	19-39
Fair	73-83	41-44	5-7	2-4	15-19	23-26	2383-2842	1198-1316	20-51	6-18
Poor	≤ 72	≤ 40	≤ 4	≤ 1	≤ 14	≤ 22	≤ 2382	≤ 1197	≤ 19	≤ 5

Interpreting the One-Leg Stance Using Mean Scores (Seconds)

The following values represent mean times based on the best of two trials conducted. Interpretation will simply categorize clients as above or below the mean values (i.e., given the lack of evidence upon which to base a more detailed Health Benefit Rating).

Age Group	Eyes Open MALE	Eyes Open FEMALE	Eyes Closed MALE	Eyes Closed FEMALE
18-39	44.4	45.0	16.9	13.1
40-49	41.6	42.1	12.0	13.5
50-59	41.5	40.9	8.6	7.9
60-69	33.8	30.4	5.1	3.6

Source: CSEP-PATH Physical Activity Training for Health Resource Manual, 2013. Reprinted with permission from the Canadian Society for Exercise Physiology.

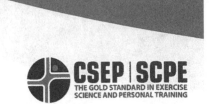

CSEP | SCPE
THE GOLD STANDARD IN EXERCISE
SCIENCE AND PERSONAL TRAINING

CSEP-PATH: EVALUATION SUMMARY REPORT - YOUTH

Client Name:	CSEP Professional:
Date (dd/mm/yr):	Location:

1. CSEP-PATH: PHYSICAL ACTIVITY & SEDENTARY BEHAVIOUR QUESTIONNAIRE (PASB-Q): YOUTH 12-17 YEARS

Health Benefit Ratings	Excellent	Very Good	Good	Fair	Poor
Total Physical Activity: *(minutes/day)*	☐ 120+	☐ 90 - 119	☐ 60 - 89	☐ 30 - 59	☐ 0 - 29
Vigorous Aerobic Activity: *(times/week)*	☐ 6+	☐ 4 - 5	☐ 3	☐ 1 - 2	☐ 0
Strength Activity: *(times/week)*	☐ 6+	☐ 4 - 5	☐ 3	☐ 1 - 2	☐ 0
Perceived Aerobic Fitness:	☐	☐	☐	☐	☐
Sedentary Behaviour: *(hours/day)*	☐ <2	☐ 2 - 4	☐ 4 - 6	☐ 6 - 8	☐ >8

2. FANTASTIC LIFESTYLE CHECKLIST

Health Benefit Ratings	Excellent	Very Good	Good	Fair	Poor
Overall Score:	☐ 85 - 100	☐ 70 - 84	☐ 55 - 69	☐ 35 - 54	☐ 0 - 54

Noted Items:

3. BODY COMPOSITION: UNDER 20 YEARS

Health Risk Ratings	Least	Increased	High	Very High	Extremely High
Body Mass Index (BMI):	☐ Normal Weight	☐ Risk of overweight	☐ Overweight/Thin	☐ Obese	☐ Severely obese/ Severely thin

4. AEROBIC FITNESS

Health Benefit Ratings	Excellent	Very Good	Good	Fair	Poor
Estimated VO$_2$max: *(ml·kg⁻¹·min⁻¹)*					

5. MUSCULOSKELETAL FITNESS

Health Benefit Ratings	Excellent	Very Good	Good	Fair	Poor
Grip Strength (kg):					
Push-ups (#):					
Sit & Reach (cm):					
Vertical jump (watts):					
Back Extension (seconds):					

	Score (seconds)
One-leg Stance – Eyes Open (sec):	
One-leg Stance – Eyes Closed (sec):	

HEALTH BENEFIT RATINGS SUMMARY

The CSEP-PATH assessment results are presented in terms of the Health Benefit Ratings calculated for each of the physical activity, sedentary behavior, lifestyle and fitness assessments.

Health Benefit Ratings	Associated Health Benefits and Risks	General Recommendation
Excellent	Optimal health benefits	Keep up the good work! What are your long-term physical activity goals? What do you plan to do to keep yourself on-track to achieve them?
Very Good	Considerable health benefits	Keep up the good work! What are your specific short- and long-term physical activity goals? What are you planning to do to achieve your goals to help you stay active for life?
Good	Many health benefits	What are your specific short- and long-term physical activity goals? What are you planning to do to achieve your goals and become more physically active?
Fair	Some health benefits, but also some risks	What are your short-term physical activity goals? What are you planning to do to achieve those goals, and then progress further from there?
Poor	Considerable health risks	What are your short-term goals to begin building physical activity into your daily life? (Evidence shows that starting with small changes and building on your successes is the best way to go.) What are you planning to do to achieve your goals?

CANADIAN PHYSICAL ACTIVITY GUIDELINES

Adults (18-64 years): For health benefits, accumulate at least 150 minutes per week of moderate-to-vigorous intensity physical activity, in bouts of 10 minutes or more. It is also beneficial to add muscle and bone strengthening activities at least 2 days per week. More daily physical activity provides greater health benefits.

Older Adults (65 years and older): For health benefits and to improve functional abilities, accumulate at least 150 minutes of moderate-to vigorous-intensity aerobic physical activity per week, in bouts of 10 minutes or more. It is also beneficial to add muscle

and bone strengthening activities using major muscle groups, at least 2 days per week. Those with poor mobility should perform physical activities to enhance balance and prevent falls.

Children (5-11 years) and Youth (12-17 years): For health benefits, accumulate at least 60 minutes of moderate-to-vigorous intensity physical activity daily. This should include: vigorous-intensity activities at least 3 days per week; and activities that strengthen muscle and bone at least 3 days per week. More daily physical activity provides greater health benefits.

Source: CSEP-PATH Physical Activity Training for Health Resource Manual, 2013. Reprinted with permission from the Canadian Society for Exercise Physiology.

☞ Look in the Book, pp. 428-429

WORKSHEET

15.3 Design a Personal Fitness and Wellness Program

You are now ready to design a fitness program to meet your own personal needs. As a guide, use one of the templates shown here, depending on your fitness goals (health-related fitness or performance-related fitness).

Name: _____

Date: _____

MISSION: Apply the F.I.T.T. principle and other training principles (found in Chapter 15 of your textbook) to design an eight-week program to suit your particular needs. Re-appraise after the eight weeks to determine improvements you have made in your fitness. The table below is for those who wish to achieve an overall improvement in their health and fitness, beginning at whatever level they find themselves. The table on the following page is for more experienced athletes who wish to design a performance-level fitness regime.

Weeks 1-8		Weeks 9-16	
Aerobic	Anaerobic (Resistance)	Aerobic	Anaerobic (Resistance)

Sample Training Program for Health-Related Fitness			
Frequency			
Intensity			
Type			
Time			

	Weeks 1-8		Weeks 9-16	
	Aerobic	Anaerobic (Resistance)	Aerobic	Anaerobic (Resistance)

Sample Training Program for Performance-Related Fitness				
Frequency				
Intensity				
Type				
Time				

Chapter 15 Quiz

The two sets of questions below will test your knowledge and broaden your understanding of the material covered in Chapter 15. Complete each set of questions according to your teacher's instructions.

Name: _____

Date: _____

Question Set 1: Training Principles and Methods and Factors Affecting Training

Multiple-Choice Questions

MISSION: Circle the letter beside the answer that you believe to be correct.

1. The acronym F.I.T.T.
   (a) is widely used in fitness and sport
   (b) describes the four basic elements of any good exercise or training plan
   (c) stands for frequency, intensity, type, and time (or duration) of training
   (d) all of the above

2. The most common way to determine one's intensity range for aerobic exercise is to compute
   (a) first the Maximal Heart Rate (MHR) and then the Target Heart Rate (THR)
   (b) first the Target Heart Rate (THR) and then the Maximal Heart Rate (MHR)
   (c) the Heart Rate Reserve
   (d) the Resting Heart Rate

3. The principle of diminishing returns is based on the fact that the improvements you gain with training
   (a) will reflect the fact that every athlete is unique
   (b) will reflect your prior level of training
   (c) will reflect the level of commitment to training
   (d) will reflect whether detraining occurs

4. Developing an overall training plan divided into distinct training periods to maximize performances at peak times is known as
   (a) sprints
   (b) high speed, explosive movements
   (c) long-distance running
   (d) periodization

5. Core training involves
   (a) the muscles that brace and stabilize your spine
   (b) the muscles of the back and abdominals
   (c) the upper limb muscles
   (d) Both (a) and (b) are correct.

6. Plyometrics training is a form of
   (a) flexibility training to decrease stress on joints
   (b) resistance training for strength and power
   (c) cardiorespiratory training to boost endurance
   (d) speed/ability/quickness training

Short-Answer Questions

MISSION: Briefly answer the following questions in the space provided:

1. What are five principles underlying all sound training programs?

2. Which two general concepts should be kept in mind when devising a training plan?

3. What factors help combat fatigue in an athlete?

Essay Questions

MISSION: On a separate piece of paper, develop a 100-word response to the following questions.

1. Summarize the ingredients of a good training program and provide examples of training principles and methods in action. (Mention components identified by Canadian Sport for Life's Long-Term Athlete Development Program that help prevent overtraining.)

2. Explain the three phases of a good cardiorespiratory training program.

3. Discuss various ways in which environmental factors can have an impact on training.

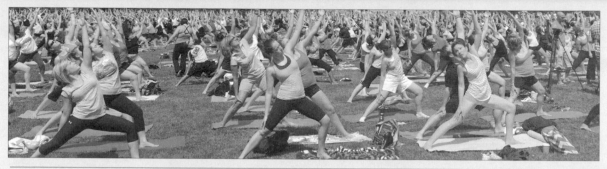

Paul McKinnon/Shutterstock

Question Set 2: Designing an Individualized Training Program

Multiple-Choice Questions

MISSION: Circle the letter beside the answer that you believe to be correct.

1. A person's fitness and training goals could include
   (a) gaining muscle strength and losing weight
   (b) preparing for an elite competition
   (c) attaining a personal best in a recreational sport
   (d) all of the above

2. A safe and effective training program features both
   (a) a continuous and an interval segment
   (b) a 40-metre dash and a walk-run test
   (c) an aerobic and an anaerobic segment
   (d) an agility and a coordination segment

3. In the aerobic segment of a training program, the participant and trainer must
   (a) monitor heart rate and perceived exertion
   (b) check muscle tightness and joint soreness
   (c) provide adequate relief between sets/exercises
   (d) all of the above

4. The 2013 CSEP-PATH manual provides the latest information on
   (a) physical activity, sedentary behaviour, and fitness levels
   (b) brain research and cognitive functioning
   (c) health-related behaviour change
   (d) (a) and (c) above

5. The 5 As of CSEP's Physical Activity Training for Health (CSEP-PATH) are
   (a) ask, appraise, analyze, alter, and accredit
   (b) ask, alert, avoid, administer, achieve
   (c) ask, answer, allow, act, adapt
   (d) ask, assess, advise, agree, assist/arrange

6. The frequency of both aerobic and anaerobic training for health-related fitness should be
   (a) once a week
   (b) three times a week
   (c) twice a week
   (d) six times a week

Short-Answer Questions

MISSION: Briefly answer the following questions in the space provided:

1. Outline the three stages involved in developing a sound individualized training program.

2. What are the benefits of warming up and cooling down during each segment of a training program?

3. List six components of fitness for which there are standardized fitness appraisals.

Essay Questions

MISSION: On a separate piece of paper, develop a 100-word response to the following questions.

1. Which factors determine what to assess and which fitness assessments are most appropriate in designing a sample training program?

2. Design a safe and effective personal anaerobic training program to suit an individual in a sport of your choice.

3. Summarize how the CSEP-PATH Resource Manual supports certified personal trainers and other exercise professionals.

WORKSHEET

My Notes on Chapter 15

Use the space below to make notes on the questions on the facing page, to record any thoughts and ideas you have on this chapter, and to store study tips to help you prepare for tests and exams.

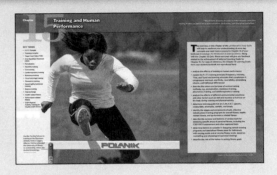

Chapter 15 Review (Student Textbook page 431)

Knowledge

1. What is the difference between training your body to perform a skill as opposed to learning a skill?

2. Describe how you could increase the intensity of (a) a cardiorespiratory training session and (b) a resistance training session and provide examples.

3. Draw a concept map that features at least six environmental factors that affect training. For each factor, show point-form information detailing how each factor impacts performance. Also include point-form information describing ways in which athletes can reduce any risks associated with each factor.

4. Besides environmental conditions, list other key physiological and psychological factors to be taken into account when developing a training schedule.

5. Create a brief fact sheet listing the criteria and procedures for establishing a safe and effective individualized training program.

6. Why are warming up and cooling down considered essential segments of any training session?

7. Compare and contrast health-related fitness and performance-related fitness.

8. Describe the components of a personalized training program that would benefit an older, overweight family member who has been inactive for some time. Be specific in your answer.

Thinking and Inquiry

9. In your notebook, make a simple visual glossary (with clear labels and definitions) to help you remember the terminology for all of the training principles and methods you learned about in Chapter 15. You may use stick figures in your drawings if you wish.

10. Which of the training principles accounts for why two athletes who participate in exactly the same training may not improve their performance to the same extent? Explain your answer.

11. Why is it important for athletes at all levels to align their training regimen with Canadian Sport for Life's Long-Term Athlete Development Model and with S.M.A.R.T. goal setting?

12. Choose an activity or a sport and plan the preparation segment, aerobic segment, resistance segment, and cool-down segment for a sample training session for that activity or sport.

13. A friend is anxious to start an individualized training program by beginning an independently developed regimen immediately. What recommendations and cautions could you give your friend to ensure safety and success?

14. Think of your favourite activity or sport. Identify which fitness tests might help improve your performance in that activity or sport.

15. Select an Olympic athlete and research their personalized training program. Present your findings in a format of your choice.

Communication

16. Interview a coach in your school or community about the risks of overtraining or under-recovery. Summarize the coach's most effective strategies for ensuring sufficient recovery and avoiding injuries and burnout. Present your findings to the class in a brief report.

17. Create a checklist of do's and don'ts that anyone could use when designing the aerobic and resistance training segments of a training program.

18. Explain to a friend or family member why it is important to have a fitness assessment performed by a properly trained and qualified individual.

Application

19. Choose a physical activity or sport in which you have been involved or one in which you would like to become involved. Apply the F.I.T.T. principle and the five principles that complement F.I.T.T. to draw up a weekly training schedule that suits your needs. Detail the specific training methods that you wish to try out. Be sure to keep safety guidelines in mind and ask your coach or teacher to approve your training schedule before you begin.

20. Define personalized training/fitness goals for yourself based on specific desired outcomes. Consult a qualified trainer or physical education teacher to ensure your goals are safe, appropriate, and attainable.

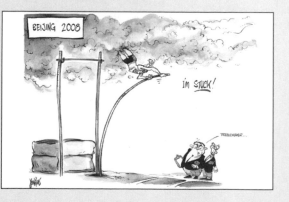

Air quality in large cities is a concern for active individuals. Beijing, for example, introduced major traffic restrictions and other measures during the 2008 Olympics in an effort to improve the air quality for athletes. (Anthony Jenkins/The Globe and Mail)

16

Ergogenic Substances and Techniques

KEY TERMS

- Ergogenic aids
- Dietary supplements
- Protein and amino acid supplements
- Caffeine
- World Anti-Doping Agency (WADA)
- Pharmacological aids
- Physiological aids
- Technological aids
- Computational fluid dynamics
- Nanotechnology

Sprinter Ben Johnson (on the right) won the gold medal at the 1988 Summer Olympics in Seoul, South Korea. He was later stripped of his gold medal and world record after he tested positive for steroids. Johnson was banned from competition for life.

AP Photo/Gary Kemper

> **"It is exercise alone that supports the spirits and keeps the mind in vigour."**
> — Cicero (106-43 BCE), Roman orator and statesman.

The exercises in this chapter of the *Lab Manual & Study Guide* will help to reinforce your understanding of some key concepts and main topics covered in Chapter 16 of your textbook *Kinesiology: An Introduction to Exercise Science*. Along with the Chapter 16 Quiz, these exercises will give you feedback related to the achievement of selected Learning Goals for Chapter 16. For ease of reference, the Chapter 16 Learning Goals from your student textbook are reproduced here:

- analyze the effects of various performance-enhancing methods and substances on human performance
- describe three basic forms of performance-enhancing substances, or ergogenic aids (nutritional, pharmacological, and physiological aids)
- identify the basic subgroups of nutritional aids (vitamins and minerals; proteins and amino acid supplements; carnitine; creatine; and caffeine)
- assess the benefits and risks related to ingestion of sport foods and energy drinks to enhance performance
- identify the basic subgroups of pharmacological aids (pain-masking drugs, anabolic steroids, prohormones, human growth hormone, and erythropoietin)
- describe drug-testing protocols used in competitive sports
- describe the role of the World Anti-Doping Agency (WADA) and its Prohibited List in fighting drug use in sport
- describe the use of physiological aids such as blood doping and drug masking
- describe the repercussions of using banned or illegal substances to enhance performance
- describe the role of computational fluid dynamics in designing clothing for speed-based sports
- describe ergogenic technologies such as "smart clothing," new reactive materials, impact sensors for helmets, and design of sports equipment based on nanotechnology
- analyze how digital innovations can boost performance

16.1 The Effects of Ergogenic Substances and Techniques

When the rewards of winning take precedent over the principle of fair play, athletes may resort to banned substances and techniques to improve their performance. Many ergogenic aids pose serious health risks, however.

Name: _____

Date: _____

MISSION: Use the space provided in the table below to briefly identify and describe the use and effects, as well as any health risks associated with the substances or techniques listed in the first column.

Type of Ergogenic Substance	Use and Effects	Health Risks
Anabolic agents		
Diuretics		
Narcotics		
Stimulants		

Type of Ergogenic Substance	Use and Effects	Health Risks
Prohormones		
Human growth hormone (HGH)		
Blood doping		
Pain-masking drugs		
Beta-blockers		
Erythropoietin (EPO)		

16.2 Technological Innovation in Sport

The invention of new sports equipment and materials can enhance athletic performance. However, just as for physiological ergogenic aids, there can be disadvantages associated with ergogenic aids based on technology.

Name: _____

Date: _____

MISSION: In the table below and on the next page, briefly describe some equipment innovations and any criticism or drawbacks associated with the items or devices listed in the first column, doing research as required. Then, choose two pieces of equipment, devices, or materials related to other sports or physical activities that are of interest to you and fill in the required information on the next page. A sample entry is provided below.

	Equipment Innovations	Criticism/Drawbacks
Hockey stick	Early North American wood sticks; more advanced wood/fibreglass design; graphite sticks	Hockey "purists" say graphite offers less control; too much curve in blade leads to poor shooting technique
Tennis racquet		
Soccer ball		
Swimsuits		
Athletic shoes		
Track surfaces		
Smartphone apps such as "Map My Run"®		

	Equipment Innovations	Criticism/Drawbacks
Bicycles		
Table tennis balls		
Artificial turf		
Hockey helmets		
Bobsleds		
"Smart" clothing		
Wireless activity trackers		

WORSHEET

Chapter 16 Quiz

The two sets of questions below will test your knowledge and broaden your understanding of the material covered in Chapter 16. Complete each set of questions according to your teacher's instructions.

Name: _____

Date: _____

Question Set 1: Nutritional, Pharmacological, and Physiological Aids

Multiple-Choice Questions

MISSION: Circle the letter beside the answer that you believe to be correct.

1. Substances and techniques used by athletes to improve performance and recovery are known as
   (a) ergogenic aids
   (b) dietary aids
   (c) physiological aids
   (d) pharmacological aids

2. Which of the following substances have athletes used to promote fat loss?
   (a) carnitine
   (b) protein supplements
   (c) creatine
   (d) caffeine

3. The international standard that identifies substances and methods that are banned in sport is known as
   (a) the World Anti-Doping Agency List
   (b) the IOC Banned List
   (c) the Canada Vigilance Program List
   (d) the Prohibited List

4. Competitors in endurance sports such as cycling may try to enhance their performance by taking
   (a) anabolic steroids
   (b) erythropoietin
   (c) beta-blockers
   (d) human growth hormone

5. Which of the following ergogenic techniques does not involve ingesting a substance?
   (a) drug masking
   (b) creatine
   (c) blood doping
   (d) human growth hormone

6. Which of the following ergogenic aids is used, illegally, by athletes to enhance aerobic athletic performance?
   (a) blood doping
   (b) creatine
   (c) erythropoietin
   (d) a and c

Short-Answer Questions

MISSION: Briefly answer the following questions in the space provided:

1. Which common stimulant, although legal, might cause problems for athletes, and why?

2. What are anabolic steroids and why do some athletes ingest them?

3. What are the side effects of ingesting extra human growth hormone (HGH)?

Essay Questions

MISSION: On a separate piece of paper, develop a 100-word response to the following questions.

1. Choose one ergogenic aid from each classification (nutritional, pharmacological, and physiological). Describe the benefits and/or risks associated with each of them.

2. Discuss drug-testing protocols in competitive sports. What are the consequences of testing positive for a banned substance at a major international event?

3. What is the stance of Health Canada and the Dietitians of Canada regarding consumption of sport foods and energy drinks?

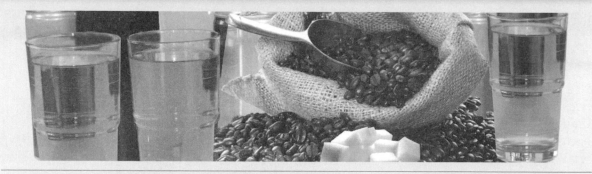

Question Set 2: Technology, Equipment Design, and Digital Aids

Multiple-Choice Questions

MISSION: Circle the letter beside the answer that you believe to be correct.

1. Today, the most significant influence on technological aids to boost athletic performance is
   (a) material science and design
   (b) aerospace engineering
   (c) digital advances
   (d) nanotechnology

2. A subfield of physics called computational fluid dynamics is now indispensable to the design of
   (a) helmets
   (b) fishing rods
   (c) basketball and training shoes
   (d) clothing for speed-based sports such as cycling, skating, and swimming

3. The world's top bobsled designers are now replicating the aerodynamics of
   (a) airplanes
   (b) Formula One race cars
   (c) a classic teardrop, airfoil shape
   (d) bodywork designed for straight-line speed

4. Protective gear made of new "reactive materials" that can flex and move with a body in motion but harden upon impact is the result of
   (a) inventions of new thermoset materials
   (b) innovations in low-friction fabric design
   (c) innovations in nanotechnology
   (d) wireless networks embedded in clothing

5. A major sport and fitness trend today is
   (a) smartphone integration with social media
   (b) wireless activity trackers
   (c) virtual gyms
   (d) all of the above

6. A tool that can measure the intensity of physical activity is
   (a) a pedometer
   (b) a health-and-fitness wristband
   (c) an accelerometer
   (d) (a) and (c) are correct

Short-Answer Questions

MISSION: Briefly answer the following questions in the space provided:

1. Give four examples of wearable fitness technology.

2. List five items of sports equipment that rely on carbon nanotubes for improved functioning.

3. What are some popular tools for measurement and motivation related to physical activity and sport?

Essay Questions

MISSION: On a separate piece of paper, develop a 100-word response to the following questions.

1. Expand on this statement: "The design and adaptation of sports and leisure products to improve performance are benefitting from a boom in technological innovation."

2. Explain, with examples, how technological innovation can lead to improved sport equipment design.

3. Discuss whether innovations in helmet design might or might not reduce the number of concussions experienced by sport participants.

My Notes on Chapter 16

Use the space below to make notes on the questions on the facing page, to record any thoughts and ideas you have on this chapter, and to store study tips to help you prepare for tests and exams.

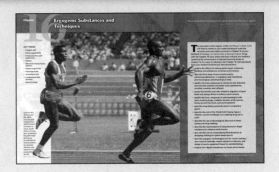

Chapter 16 Review (Student Textbook page 451)

Knowledge

1. Why should both elite and everyday athletes educate themselves about dietary supplements before deciding whether or not to take a particular product to boost performance?

2. In a table, list the risks and benefits associated with consumption of sport drinks, sport gels and bars, liquid meals, and energy drinks. Do the risks appear to outweigh the benefits, or vice versa?

3. Identify and define the two types of ergogenic aids to boost athletic performance that often involve the use of prohibited substances and methods, and give two or three examples of such aids.

4. What are the main reasons that some athletes use pharmacological aids?

5. Give some examples of how applied physics is having a positive impact on sports clothing design.

6. Describe some of the functionalities of "smart clothing" and give one example of how these innovations can enhance human performance.

7. Give three or four examples to show how nanotechnology is improving the design and function of sports equipment.

8. Give three examples of sports-related technologies that provide both "measurement and motivation."

Thinking and Inquiry

9. You have a friend who takes supplemental vitamins and minerals well in excess of recommended levels. Based on what you have learned in this chapter, what advice would you give your friend and how would you support your point of view?

10. Which individuals or organizations do you consider trustworthy and reliable sources of information about ergogenic nutritional aids, and why?

11. Despite the efforts of the World Anti-Doping Agency and the negative public backlash directed at athletes who are caught doping, why do you think some athletes continue to dope?

12. Imagine that you are a member of an Olympic team. One of your teammates has confided that he or she is considering using a substance or method currently on the Prohibited List. Develop an argument to dissuade your teammate from using this substance or method.

13. Think of a wearable fitness technology that you would like to see invented and explain how it would help improve athletic performance.

14. List some advantages and disadvantages of pressure sensors, apps, and other digital technologies that are capable of uploading your workout data to social media sites.

Communication

15. With guidance from your teacher, invite a nutritionist, dietitian, sport coach, or personal trainer to class to present their views on the use of nutritional aids to boost performance. Prepare questions in advance and be prepared to participate in the follow-up discussion.

16. Design a clear and simple information guide in a format of your choice to teach younger students about the World Anti-Doping Agency's role in restricting ergogenic aids in efforts to protect athletes' health and ensure fair play in sport.

17. As a class, discuss whether the growing prevalence of impact sensors used in helmets to monitor blows to the head might unintentionally impede efforts to restrict violence in sports.

Application

18. Contact a local coach or community sports programmer to find out which ergogenic aids are banned in your school or community, and why.

19. Which of the performance-enhancing sports fabrics, materials, clothing, or equipment described in Chapter 16 would you like to try out? How do you think these items would help to improve your own sport performance or the performance of others who might use them. Are there any risks?

20. Given the increasing popularity of computerized fitness equipment, wireless activity trackers, desktop treadmills, virtual gyms, and the like, do you think that businesses such as fitness facilities will simply disappear during your lifetime? Give plausible reasons for your answer.

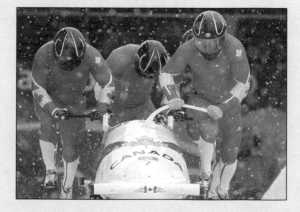

Due in part to a sleek new bobsled design based on racecar engineering, Canada won bronze in the four-man bobsled event at the 2010 Olympic Winter Games in Whistler, B.C. (CP Photo/Jeff McIntosh)

Career Choices

Investigate a career in one of the fields mentioned in this unit. Ideally, you should interview someone working within the field for this assignment. You can ask him or her the following questions and a lot more as well.

Name: _____

Date: _____

MISSION: Answer the series of questions below in relation to the career you have selected. If you interviewed a person for this career information, use quotation marks to distinguish what they said from your own comments on the career. Give the person's name and job title.

1 Career and description

_____

_____

_____

_____

_____

2 List at least two post-secondary institutions in Ontario and/or Canada that offer programs for this career.

_____

_____

_____

_____

3 Choose one of the above institutions and determine the required courses in the first year of study for this program.

_____

_____

_____

_____

4 How many years of post-secondary education are required before beginning this career? Is an internship or apprenticeship required?

_____

_____

_____

_____

5 What is the demand for individuals qualified for this occupation? If possible, provide some employment data to support your answer.

_____

_____

_____

_____

6 What is the average starting salary for this career? What is the top salary? On what do salary increases depend in this career?

_____

_____

_____

_____

7 List occupational settings where a person with these qualifications could work.

_____

_____

_____

_____

KINESIOLOGY—SAMPLE FINAL EXAM

Congratulations on completing your first course in Kinesiology!

On the next eight pages is a sample final exam based on what you have covered in this course.

This sample final exam is similar in organization and in length to the actual exam that your teacher will administer after you have had a chance to familiarize yourself with the format of a typical final examination in this subject area. To give you sufficient practice in answering various types of exam questions, including ones that require the labelling of anatomical diagrams, this sample final exam is divided into two sessions as outlined below.

Grade 12 Final Exam: Kinesiology Course

Name of School: _____

Name of Teacher: _____

Your Name: _____

Date: _____

☞ **Session 1**

Part A : Multiple-Choice Questions	30 Questions	15 Marks
Part B: True or False	20 Questions	10 Marks
Part C: Fill in the Blanks	20 Questions	10 Marks
Part D: Short-Answer Questions	5 Questions	10 Marks
Part E: Essay Question	1 Question	17 Marks

☞ **Session 2**

Part F: Anatomical Labelling	76 Labels	38 Marks

Total		_____ /100 Marks

Instructions

You will have at least 90 minutes to 2 hours to complete each session of this sample exam (this timing may vary somewhat according to your teacher's specific scheduling requirements).

You can write your rough answer to the essay question in Part E on a separate sheet of lined paper, and then transfer your clean response onto the lined page at the end of this exam (see page 288).

Be sure to fill in the name of your school, the name of your teacher, your name, and the date before you begin this sample exam.

Good luck!

Sample Final Exam: Session 1

1. Children aged five to 17 need at least
   (a) one hour of exercise per day
   (b) two hours of exercise per day
   (c) 20 minutes of exercise per day
   (d) 150 minutes of exercise per week

2. Kinesiology is the systematic study of
   (a) human sports performance
   (b) the physiological, psychological, and sociological aspects of human movement
   (c) the structure and function of the human body
   (d) human growth and development

3. The Victorians believed that sport
   (a) should be accessible to the lower classes
   (b) woud benefit a woman's delicate constitution
   (c) would strengthen a young man's character
   (d) should be organized into professional leagues

4. The years 1882-1914 saw the growth of
   (a) amateur sports only
   (b) professional sports teams only
   (c) women's professional sports
   (d) both amateur and professional sports

5. A commercial agreement by which an athlete promotes a product or service is called
   (a) an endorsement deal
   (b) a testimonial
   (c) a franchise
   (d) a player contract

6. Professional sports teams make money by
   (a) sales of replica products
   (b) sales of food and beverages at stadiums
   (c) selling advertising and broadcasting rights
   (d) all of the above

7. Gender-based inequities in sport result in
   (a) little difference in salaries and prize money for female athletes compared to male athletes
   (b) the banning of women from marathons
   (c) more drug tests for women compared to men
   (d) a power imbalance between women and men

8. The IAAF's gender test looks only at
   (a) amount of testosterone in the athlete's body
   (b) an athlete's genetic makeup
   (c) an athlete's anatomy
   (d) an athlete's body chemistry

9. The term "anterior" refers to
   (a) back surfaces of the body
   (b) front surfaces of the body
   (c) upward surfaces of the body
   (d) downward surfaces of the body

10. Which of the following is not a function of the human skeletal system?
    (a) structural support and protection
    (b) growth centre for cells
    (c) reservoir of vitamins
    (d) movement

11. Muscles that hold a joint in place so movements can occur at another joint are
    (a) agonist muscles
    (b) antagonist muscles
    (c) skeletal muscles
    (d) stabilizers

12. The point where the muscle attaches to the bone that is moved most is called
    (a) the insertion
    (b) the origin
    (c) the landmark
    (d) the tendon

13. The energy system used in powerful, relatively short-lived physical actions is known as
    (a) glycolysis
    (b) the aerobic system
    (c) cellular respiration
    (d) the anaerobic system

14. Slow-twitch muscle fibres are ideal for
    (a) short sprints
    (b) powerlifting
    (c) explosive jumping
    (d) long-distance cycling

15. Cardiac muscle cells that make up the myocardium are said to be "excitable" because
    (a) with electrical stimulation they will contract
    (b) they are similar to skeletal muscle
    (c) they are controlled involuntarily
    (d) they are found only in the heart

16. The combination of inspiration and expiration together is known as
    (a) diffusion
    (b) ventilation
    (c) breathing
    (d) the maximal rate of oxygen consumption

17. This term describes how human growth progresses first in the head, followed by the trunk, and then the extremities:
    (a) the proximodistal sequence
    (b) the critical period
    (c) the cephalocaudal sequence
    (d) peak height velocity

18. Learned sequences of voluntary movements that combine to produce an action are known as
    (a) developmental skills
    (b) manipulation skills
    (c) motor skills
    (d) locomotor skills

19. The categories of fundamental movement skills (FMS) that underlie physical literacy are
    (a) travelling, receiving, and sending
    (b) object control, balance, and landing
    (c) catching, striking, and dribbling
    (d) stability, locomotion, and manipulation

Multiple Choice (Continued)

20. Resistance to a change in motion is known as
   (a) inertia
   (b) friction
   (c) gravity
   (d) mass

21. Torque is the rotary effect created by
   (a) a centric force
   (b) a ground reaction force
   (c) a frictional force
   (d) an eccentric (off-centre) force

22. Human movement is usually a combination of
   (a) internal forces acting together
   (b) Newton's laws acting together
   (c) rotations of individual body segments
   (d) linear and rotational motion

23. The greater the applied impulse, the greater
   (a) the increase in momentum
   (b) the increase in acceleration
   (c) the increase in force
   (d) the increase in velocity

24. Angular momentum is constant when
   (a) an object is part of a dynamic system
   (b) an object is part of a static system
   (c) an object is in a state of equilibrium
   (d) an object is free in the air

25. Inefficient movements can lead to
   (a) an energy leak
   (b) increased fatigue
   (c) reduced energy output
   (d) all of the above

26. Your estimated resting metabolic rate affects
   (a) your daily caloric need
   (b) your daily rest and recovery needs
   (c) your daily protein requirements
   (d) your daily physical activity level

27. Reflex dilation of skin results in
   (a) fluid loss
   (b) electroyte imbalance
   (c) heating of the body
   (d) cooling of the body

28. Resistance training is also known as
   (a) endurance training
   (b) plyometrics training
   (c) strength training
   (d) base training

29. The training principle that relies on the body's gradual adaptation to greater stresses is
   (a) diminishing returns
   (b) progressive overload
   (c) specificity
   (d) reversibility

30. Morphine and heroin are examples of
   (a) cannabinoids
   (b) anabolic agents
   (c) drug-masking agents
   (d) pain-masking drugs

Part B: True or False (10 Marks)

MISSION: Indicate with a "T" or "F" whether the following statements are True or False.

1.	Research on the positive effects of physical activity on cognitive functioning is inconclusive.	
2.	One-quarter of Canadians are not active at the levels recommended for good health.	
3.	Lifestyle diseases are related to the twin problems of inactivity and obesity.	
4.	The ancient Romans developed the sporting events that formed the early Olympic Games.	
5.	Values related to physical activity and sport are unrelated to societal values as a whole.	
6.	A major contribution of Aboriginal peoples to Canadian and international sport is lacrosse.	
7.	The Winter and Summer Olympic Games are amateurs-only events.	
8.	Up to 96 percent of an athlete's earnings can come from endorsement fees.	
9.	Seniors and overweight people are rarely misled when it comes to health and wellness products .	
10.	Professional sport has long been regarded as the "last closet" in terms of sexual orientation.	
11.	The axial skeleton includes the movable limbs and their supporting structures.	
12.	The neuromuscular system depends on interactions between nerves and muscles.	
13.	Fats play the central role in providing energy for use by cells in our bodies.	
14.	Arterioles enable the exchange of gases and nutrients between the blood and the tissues.	
15.	Cardiac output (Q) is the volume of blood pumped out of the left ventricle in one hour.	
16.	Few factors in addition to chronological age affect human growth and development.	
17.	Motor learning involves a combination of physical and psychological factors.	
18.	A proficient movement pattern maximizes energy expenditure while facilitating performance.	
19.	How stable a person is while performing a physical task depends only on the person's base of support.	
20.	Movement usually occurs in the direction of the applied force.	

Part C: Fill in the Blanks (10 Marks)

MISSION: Write in the missing word or words to complete each sentence below.

1. Fatty plaque buildup on the walls of the coronary arteries can eventually lead to a _____.

2. _____ serves as an indicator of overall cardiovascular health.

3. Principles that recognize and respect the varying developmental needs of children are at the heart of the _____ model.

4. The ability to apply a skill learned in the context of one activity to a different activity is known as skill _____.

5. A highly focussed mental state that is conducive to top performance is known as a(n) _____ performance state.

6. Newton's second law of motion is also known as the law of _____.

7. The design of equipment and devices to assist the human body in the performance of everyday tasks is known as _____.

8. Stability depends on four factors: _____, _____, _____, and _____.

9. The production of maximum _____ requires the use of all possible joint movements that contribute to a task's objective.

10. _____ is the amount of rotation that a spinning object undergoes per unit of time.

11. Movement that is a product of the world we live in is known as _____ movement.

12. Found in gram amounts in food, _____ include carbohydrates, proteins, and fats.

13. The female athlete triad has three components: low energy availability, menstrual irregularities, and low _____ mass.

14. Athletes and active individuals need to ensure _____ meals and snacks throughout the day in order to supply the required amounts of energy and nutrients to the body.

15. _____ is a life-threatening condition that occurs when there is a complete failure of the body's heat-regulatory system.

16. _____ training involves the muscles of the back and abdominals and is a key component of most training programs.

17. Every effective training program must allow time for _____ and _____.

18. Physiological test results are a necessary preliminary to designing training programs for both health-related fitness and _____ fitness.

19. The CSEP-PATH assessment and training procedures allow accredited exercise professionals to design a _____ fitness program to suit each client.

20. Another word for "performance-enhancing" is _____.

Part D: Short-Answer Questions (10 Marks)

MISSION: Provide short answers to the following questions.

1. List four factors contributing to the physical inactivity crisis, and suggest four ways to overcome sedentarism and other barriers to physical activity.

2. Identify some historical events and pioneers in the removal of gender stereotyping, racial barriers, and discrimination based on sexual orientation in sport and physical activity.

3. List three ways in which professional sport has become a "big business" in today's world.

4. Identify four prevalent ethical issues related to sport and physical activity today.

5. What is meant by the Long-Term Athlete Development (LTAD) model?

Part E: Essay Question (17 Marks)

MISSION: Answer any **one** of the following questions in paragraph format (write three or four paragraphs for th essay question).

1. Explain the important roles of families, schools, communities, and government in promoting lifelong physical literacy for all Canadians.

2. Discuss ways in which individuals can maintain healthy body systems and a healthy body weight and supply their bodies with sufficient energy each day.

3. Describe the cardiovascular system's response to exercise, including the effects of training on this body system.

4. Explain the essential factors that determine healthy human growth and development, including the physical, social, and mental health benefits of participation in physical activity and/ or sport.

5. Explain the various ways in which knowledge of biomechanical concepts and principles can be applied to improve human performance, reduce the risk of injury, and facilitate rehabilitation following illness or disruption of a movement pattern.

6. If you were coaching athletes at different developmental levels, what approaches and strategies, including mental fitness activities, would you implement to help optimize each athlete's performance?

7. Compare and contrast legal versus illegal ergogenic aids that athletes in a particular sport can use to enhance their performance.

Part F: Anatomical Labelling (38 Marks)

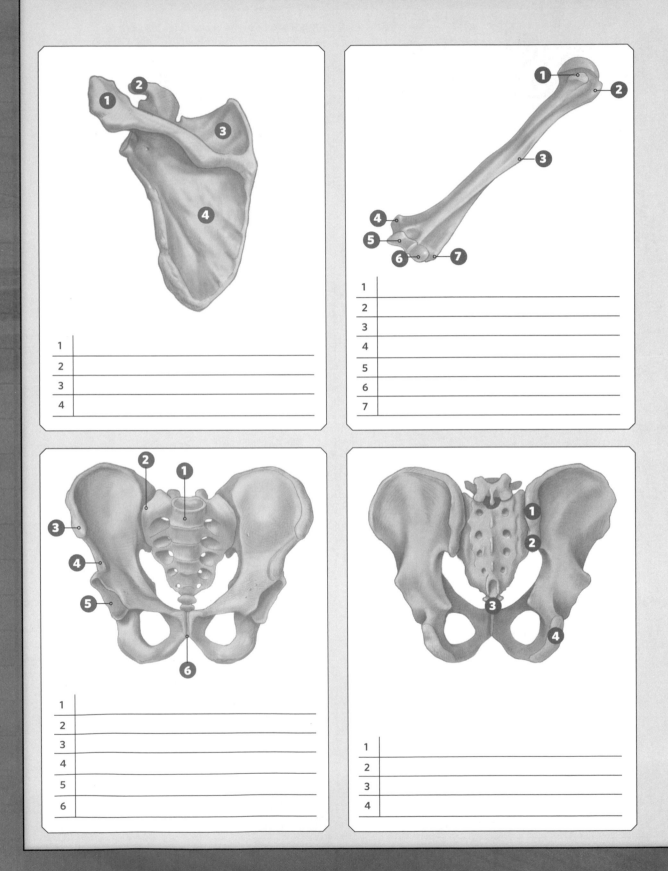

1 _____
2 _____
3 _____
4 _____

1 _____
2 _____
3 _____
4 _____
5 _____
6 _____
7 _____

1 _____
2 _____
3 _____
4 _____
5 _____
6 _____

1 _____
2 _____
3 _____
4 _____

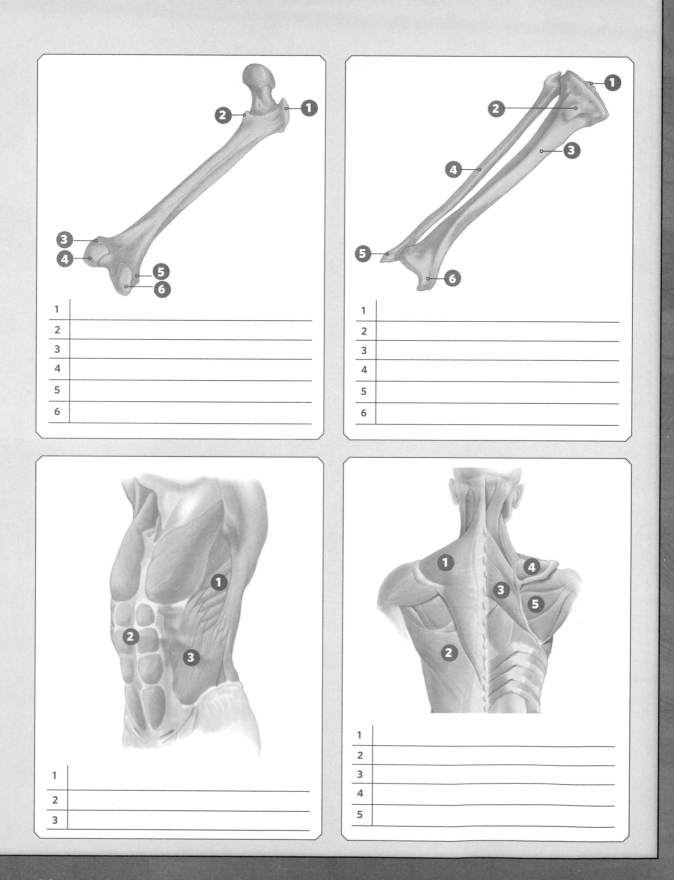

1 _____
2 _____
3 _____
4 _____
5 _____
6 _____

1 _____
2 _____
3 _____
4 _____
5 _____
6 _____

1 _____
2 _____
3 _____

1 _____
2 _____
3 _____
4 _____
5 _____

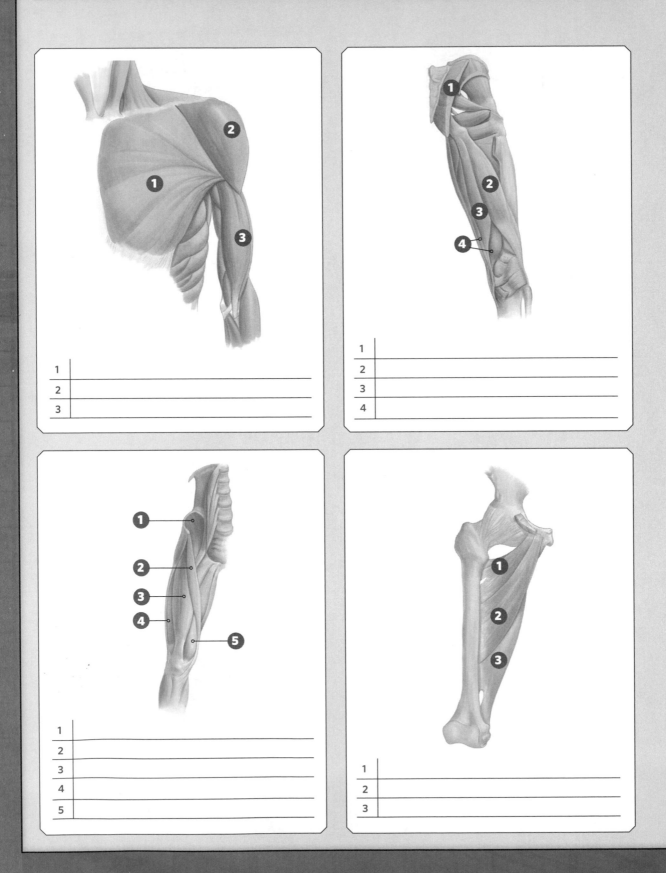

1 _____
2 _____
3 _____

1 _____
2 _____
3 _____
4 _____

1 _____
2 _____
3 _____
4 _____
5 _____

1 _____
2 _____
3 _____

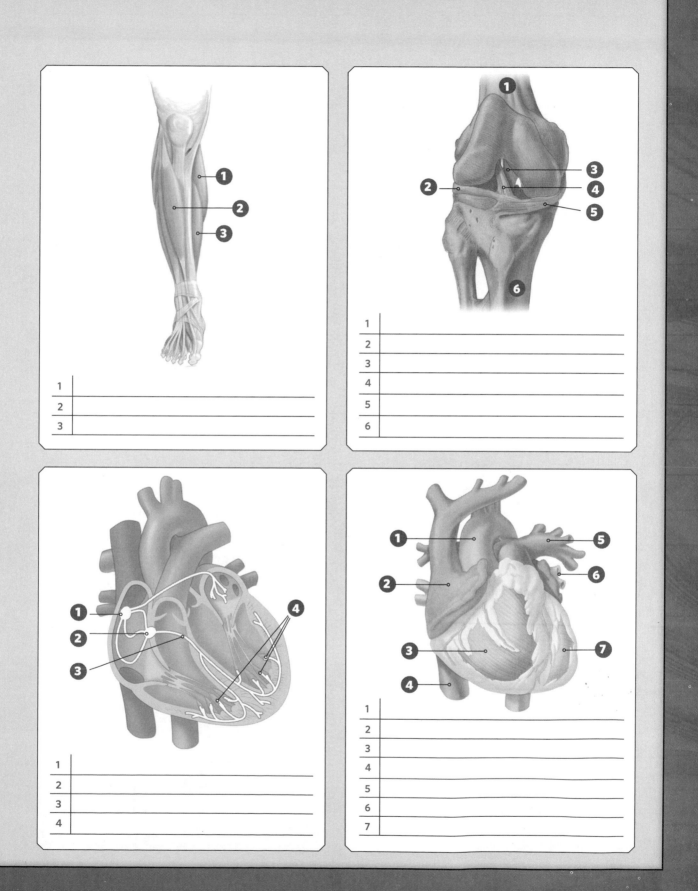

1 _____
2 _____
3 _____

1 _____
2 _____
3 _____
4 _____
5 _____
6 _____

1 _____
2 _____
3 _____
4 _____

1 _____
2 _____
3 _____
4 _____
5 _____
6 _____
7 _____

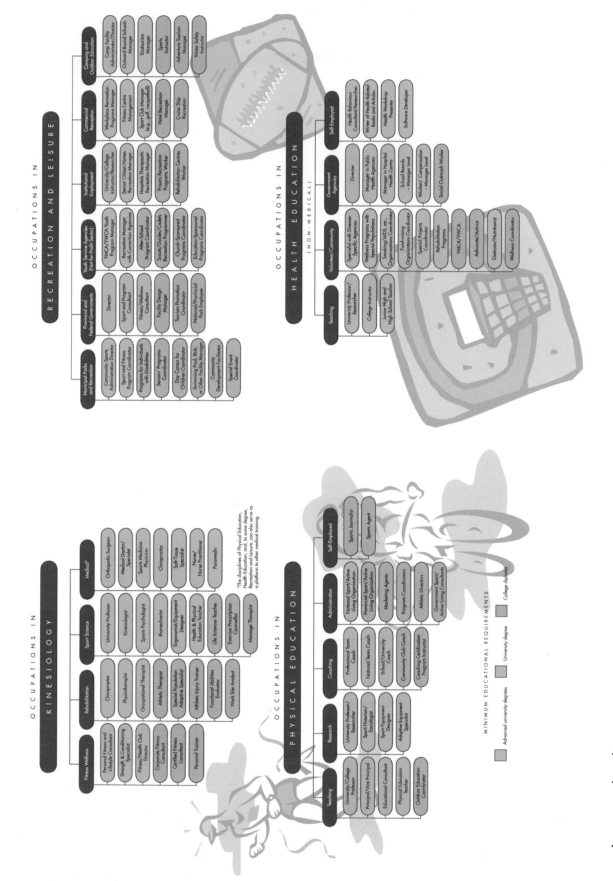

OCCUPATIONS IN RECREATION AND LEISURE

Municipal Parks and Recreation
- Community Sports Administration Director
- Sport and Fitness Program Coordinator
- Programs for Individuals with Disabilities
- Seniors' Programs Coordinator
- Day Camps for Children Coordinator
- Swimming Pool, Rink or Other Facility Manager
- Community Development Facilitator
- Special Event Coordinator

Provincial and Federal Governments
- Director
- Sport and Program Consultant
- Fitness/Wellness Consultant
- Facility Design Manager
- Tourism Promotion Coordinator
- National/Provincial Park Employee

Youth Service Agencies (Not-for-Profit Sector)
- YMCA/YWCA Youth Program Manager
- Recreation Manager with Correction Agencies
- After-School Program Coordinator
- Scouts/Guides/Cadets Recreation Programmer
- Church Sponsored Programs Coordinator
- Education-Sponsored Programs Coordinator

Institutional Employment
- University/College Instructor/Researcher
- Senior Citizen Homes Recreation Manager
- Hospitals Therapeutic Recreation Manager
- Prison Recreation Programs Worker
- Rehabilitation Centre Worker

Commercial Recreation
- Workplace Recreation Programs Manager
- Fitness Centre Management
- Sport Club Manager (e.g., golf, racquetball)
- Hotel Recreation Manager
- Cruise Ship Recreation

Camping and Outdoor Education
- Camp Facility Administrator/Director
- Outward Bound Schools Manager
- Ecotourism Manager
- Sports Instructor
- Adventure Tourism Manager
- Water Safety Instructor

OCCUPATIONS IN HEALTH EDUCATION (NON-MEDICAL)

Teaching
- University Professor/Researcher
- College Instructor
- Junior High and High School Teacher

Volunteer/Community
- Specialist with Disease Specific Agencies
- Wellness Programs with Special Populations
- Smoking/AIDS, etc. Organizations Coordinator
- Fund-raising Organizations Coordinator
- Special Projects Coordinator
- Rehabilitation Programs
- YMCA/YWCA
- Advocate/Activist
- Dietician/Nutritionist
- Wellness Coordinator

Government Agencies
- Director
- Manager in Public Health Agencies
- Manager in Hospital Health Centre
- School Boards – Manager Level
- Workers' Compensation – Manager Level
- Social Outreach Worker

Self-Employed
- Health Behaviour Consultant/Researcher
- Writer of Health-Related Books and Articles
- Health Workshop Presenter
- Software Developer

OCCUPATIONS IN KINESIOLOGY

Fitness/Wellness
- Personal Fitness and Lifestyle Consultant
- Strength & Conditioning Specialist
- Fitness/Health Club Director
- Corporate Fitness Consultant
- Certified Fitness Consultant
- Personal Trainer

Rehabilitation
- Chiropractor
- Physiotherapist
- Occupational Therapist
- Athletic Therapist
- Special Population Adaptive Specialist
- Athletic Injury Trainer
- Functional Abilities Evaluator
- Work Site Analyst

Sport Science
- University Professor
- Kinesiologist
- Sports Psychologist
- Biomechanist
- Ergonomic/Equipment Designer
- Health & Physical Education Teacher
- Life Sciences Teacher
- Exercise Prescription Counsellor
- Massage Therapist

Medical*
- Orthopedic Surgeon
- Medical Doctor/Specialist
- Sports Medicine Physician
- Chiropractor
- Soft-Tissue Specialist
- Nurse/Nurse Practitioner
- Paramedic

*The disciplines of Physical Education, Health Education, and, to some degree, Recreation and Leisure, can also serve as a platform to other medical training.

OCCUPATIONS IN PHYSICAL EDUCATION

Teaching
- University/College Professor
- Principal/Vice Principal
- Educational Consultant
- Physical Education Teacher
- Outdoor Education Coordinator

Research
- University Professor/Researcher
- Sport Historian/Sociologist
- Sport Equipment Designer
- Adaptive Equipment Specialist

Coaching
- Professional Team Coach
- National Team Coach
- School/University Coach
- Community Club Coach
- Coaching Certification Program Instructor

Administration
- National Sport/Active Living Organization
- Provincial Sport/Active Living Organization
- Marketing Agents
- Program Coordinators
- Athletic Directors
- Government Sport/Active Living Consultant

Self-Employed
- Sports Journalist
- Sports Agent

MINIMUM EDUCATIONAL REQUIREMENTS
- Advanced university degrees
- University degree
- College diploma

◆ Kinesiology — Careers Chart
© www.thompsonbooks.com

www.thompsonbooks.com

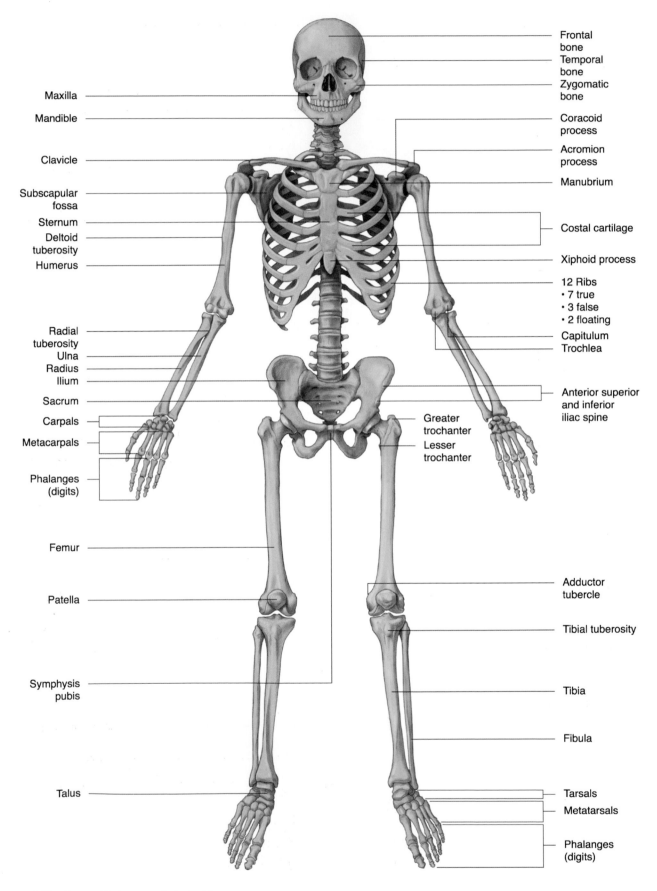

Frontal
bone

Temporal
bone

Zygomatic
bone

Maxilla

Mandible

Coracoid
process

Acromion
process

Clavicle

Manubrium

Subscapular
fossa

Sternum

Costal cartilage

Deltoid
tuberosity

Humerus

Xiphoid process

12 Ribs
• 7 true
• 3 false
• 2 floating

Radial
tuberosity

Capitulum

Ulna

Trochlea

Radius

Ilium

Sacrum

Anterior superior
and inferior
iliac spine

Carpals

Greater
trochanter

Metacarpals

Lesser
trochanter

Phalanges
(digits)

Femur

Adductor
tubercle

Patella

Tibial tuberosity

Symphysis
pubis

Tibia

Fibula

Talus

Tarsals

Metatarsals

Phalanges
(digits)

◆ The Human Skeleton — Anterior View
©www.thompsonbooks.com

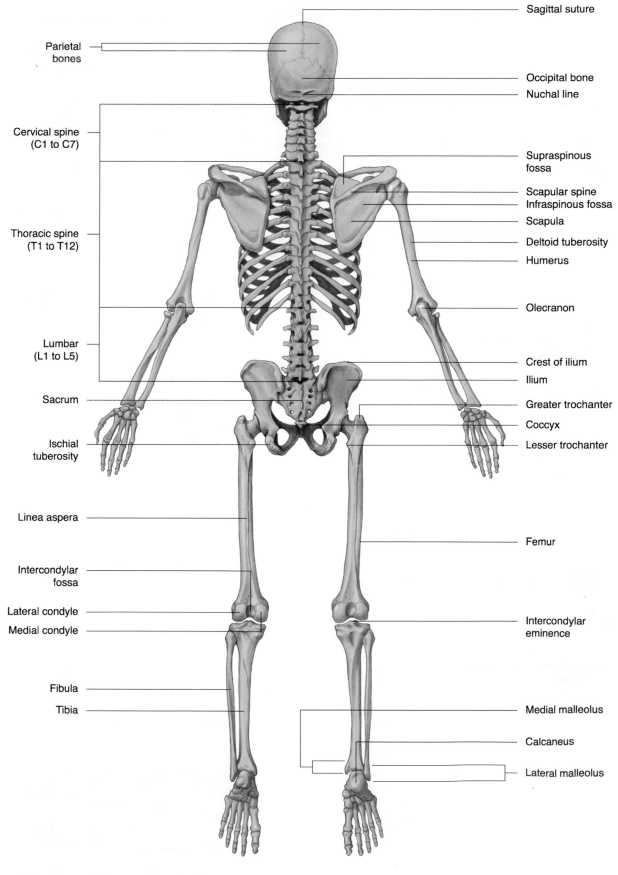

Parietal
bones

Cervical spine
(C1 to C7)

Thoracic spine
(T1 to T12)

Lumbar
(L1 to L5)

Sacrum

Ischial
tuberosity

Linea aspera

Intercondylar
fossa

Lateral condyle

Medial condyle

Fibula

Tibia

Sagittal suture

Occipital bone

Nuchal line

Supraspinous
fossa

Scapular spine

Infraspinous fossa

Scapula

Deltoid tuberosity

Humerus

Olecranon

Crest of ilium

Ilium

Greater trochanter

Coccyx

Lesser trochanter

Femur

Intercondylar
eminence

Medial malleolus

Calcaneus

Lateral malleolus

◆ The Human Skeleton — Posterior View

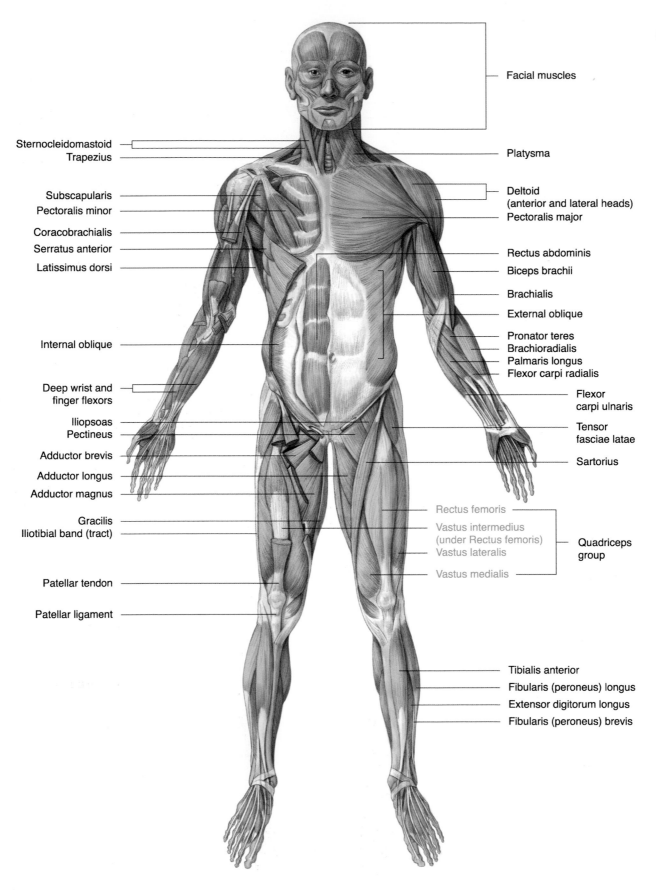

Facial muscles

Sternocleidomastoid
Trapezius

Platysma

Subscapularis
Pectoralis minor

Deltoid
(anterior and lateral heads)
Pectoralis major

Coracobrachialis
Serratus anterior
Latissimus dorsi

Rectus abdominis
Biceps brachii

Brachialis

External oblique

Internal oblique

Pronator teres
Brachioradialis
Palmaris longus
Flexor carpi radialis

Deep wrist and
finger flexors

Flexor
carpi ulnaris

Iliopsoas
Pectineus

Tensor
fasciae latae

Adductor brevis

Sartorius

Adductor longus

Adductor magnus

Rectus femoris

Gracilis
Iliotibial band (tract)

Vastus intermedius
(under Rectus femoris)
Vastus lateralis

Quadriceps
group

Vastus medialis

Patellar tendon

Patellar ligament

Tibialis anterior
Fibularis (peroneus) longus
Extensor digitorum longus
Fibularis (peroneus) brevis

◆ The Muscular System — Anterior View
© www.thompsonbooks.com

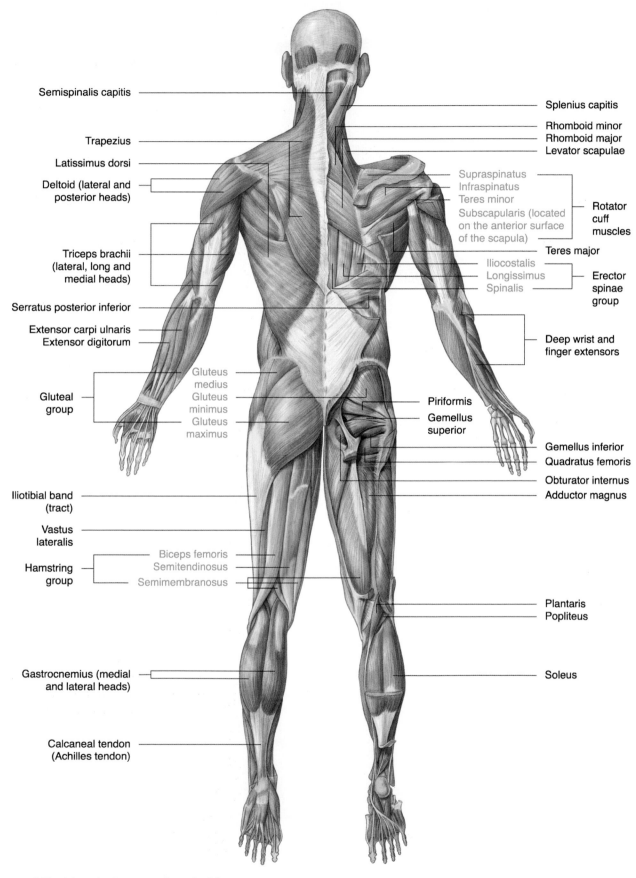

Semispinalis capitis

Trapezius

Latissimus dorsi

Deltoid (lateral and
posterior heads)

Triceps brachii
(lateral, long and
medial heads)

Serratus posterior inferior

Extensor carpi ulnaris

Extensor digitorum

Gluteal
group

Gluteus
medius
Gluteus
minimus
Gluteus
maximus

Iliotibial band
(tract)

Vastus
lateralis

Hamstring
group

Biceps femoris
Semitendinosus
Semimembranosus

Gastrocnemius (medial
and lateral heads)

Calcaneal tendon
(Achilles tendon)

Splenius capitis

Rhomboid minor
Rhomboid major
Levator scapulae

Supraspinatus
Infraspinatus
Teres minor
Subscapularis (located
on the anterior surface
of the scapula)

Rotator
cuff
muscles

Teres major

Iliocostalis
Longissimus
Spinalis

Erector
spinae
group

Deep wrist and
finger extensors

Piriformis

Gemellus
superior

Gemellus inferior

Quadratus femoris

Obturator internus

Adductor magnus

Plantaris

Popliteus

Soleus

◆ The Muscular System — Posterior View
©www.thompsonbooks.com

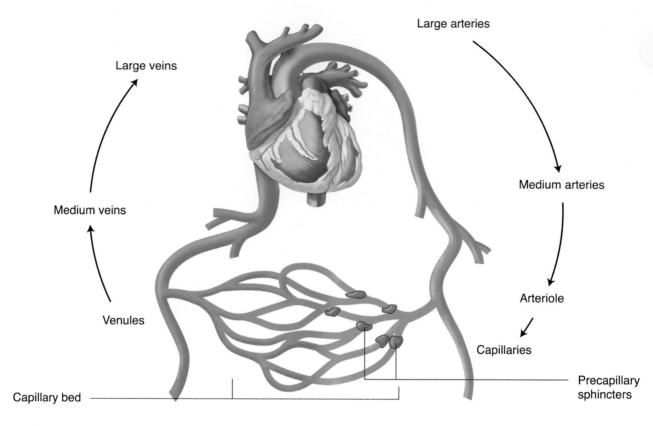

Large veins

Large arteries

Medium veins

Medium arteries

Venules

Arteriole

Capillaries

Precapillary
sphincters

Capillary bed

◆ The Vascular System (Summary)
©www.thompsonbooks.com

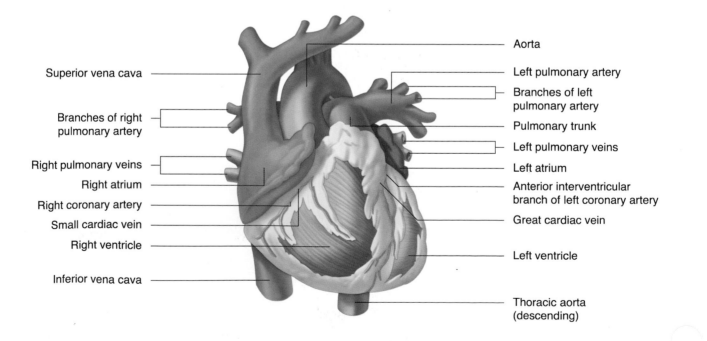

Superior vena cava

Aorta

Left pulmonary artery

Branches of left
pulmonary artery

Branches of right
pulmonary artery

Pulmonary trunk

Left pulmonary veins

Right pulmonary veins

Left atrium

Right atrium

Right coronary artery

Anterior interventricular
branch of left coronary artery

Small cardiac vein

Great cardiac vein

Right ventricle

Left ventricle

Inferior vena cava

Thoracic aorta
(descending)

◆ Coronary Vessels and Other Major Structures (Anterior View)
©www.thompsonbooks.com

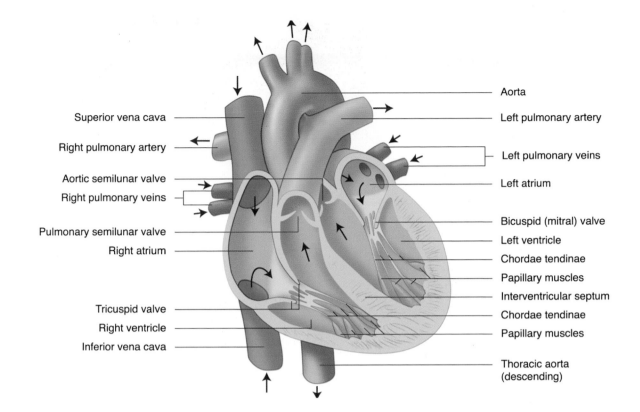

Superior vena cava

Right pulmonary artery

Aortic semilunar valve

Right pulmonary veins

Pulmonary semilunar valve

Right atrium

Tricuspid valve

Right ventricle

Inferior vena cava

Aorta

Left pulmonary artery

Left pulmonary veins

Left atrium

Bicuspid (mitral) valve

Left ventricle

Chordae tendinae

Papillary muscles

Interventricular septum

Chordae tendinae

Papillary muscles

Thoracic aorta
(descending)

◆ Anatomy of the Heart Showing the Flow of Blood
   ©www.thompsonbooks.com

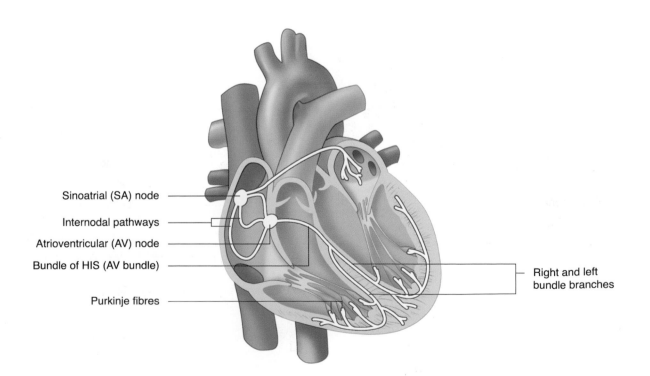

Sinoatrial (SA) node

Internodal pathways

Atrioventricular (AV) node

Bundle of HIS (AV bundle)

Purkinje fibres

Right and left
bundle branches

◆ Electrical Conduction System of the Heart
   ©www.thompsonbooks.com

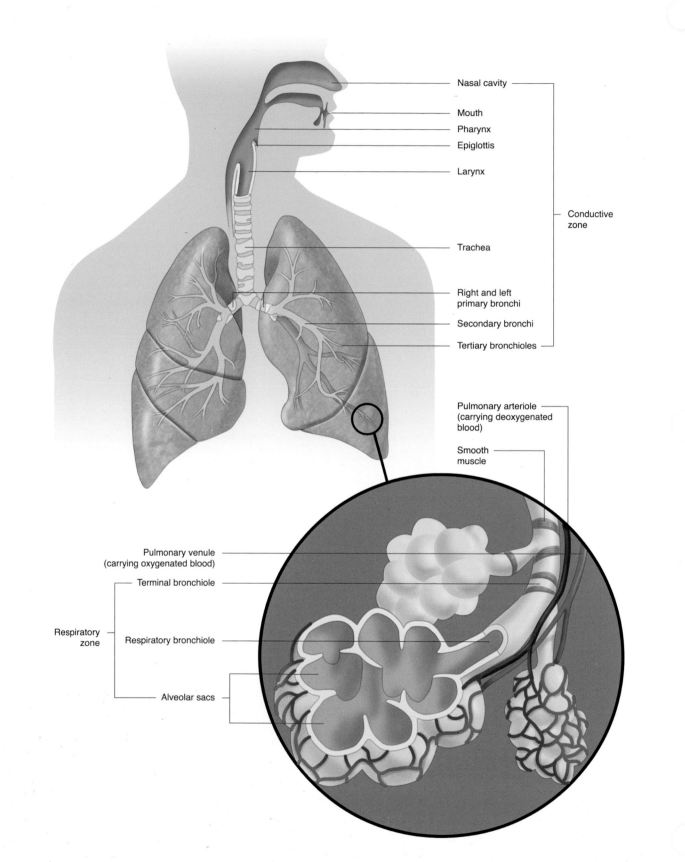

Nasal cavity

Mouth

Pharynx

Epiglottis

Larynx

Conductive zone

Trachea

Right and left primary bronchi

Secondary bronchi

Tertiary bronchioles

Pulmonary arteriole (carrying deoxygenated blood)

Smooth muscle

Pulmonary venule (carrying oxygenated blood)

Terminal bronchiole

Respiratory zone

Respiratory bronchiole

Alveolar sacs

◆ The Respiratory System
© www.thompsonbooks.com